THE SECRET PLEASURES
OF MENOPAUSE

Also by Christiane Northrup, M.D.

Books

Mother-Daughter Wisdom
The Wisdom of Menopause
The Wisdom of Menopause Journal*
Women's Bodies, Women's Wisdom

Audio/Video Programs

Creating Health
The Empowering Women Gift Collection, with Louise L. Hay;
Susan Jeffers, Ph.D.; and Caroline Myss*
Igniting Intuition, with Mona Lisa Schulz, M.D., Ph.D.*
Intuitive Listening, with Mona Lisa Schulz, M.D., Ph.D.*
Menopause and Beyond (CD and DVD available March 2010)*
Mother-Daughter Wisdom
The Power of Joy*
The Secret Pleasures of Menopause*
Women's Bodies, Women's Wisdom

Women's Wisdom Web Community

Women's Health Wisdom E-letter
Women's Wisdom Circle

Miscellaneous

Women's Bodies, Women's Wisdom Healing Cards (a 50-card deck)*
Women's Wisdom Perpetual Flip Calendar*

All of the above are available from **www.drnorthrup.com**.

*The items with an asterisk are also available from Hay House.

Please visit Hay House USA: **www.hayhouse.com**®
Hay House Australia: **www.hayhouse.com.au**
Hay House UK: **www.hayhouse.co.uk**
Hay House South Africa: **www.hayhouse.co.za**
Hay House India: **www.hayhouse.co.in**

THE SECRET PLEASURES
OF MENOPAUSE

CHRISTIANE
NORTHRUP, M.D.

in consultation with
Edward A. Taub, M.D., F.A.A.P.;
Ferid Murad, M.D., Ph.D.; and
David Oliphant

HAY HOUSE, INC.
Carlsbad, California • New York City
London • Sydney • Johannesburg
Vancouver • Hong Kong • New Delhi

Published and distributed in the United States by: Hay House, Inc.: www.hayhouse.
com • *Published and distributed in Australia by:* Hay House Australia Pty. Ltd.: www.
hayhouse.com.au • *Published and distributed in the United Kingdom by:* Hay House
UK, Ltd.: www.hayhouse.co.uk • *Published and distributed in the Republic of South
Africa by:* Hay House SA (Pty), Ltd.: www.hayhouse.co.za • *Distributed in Canada by:*
Raincoast: www.raincoast.com • *Published in India by:* Hay House Publishers India:
www.hayhouse.co.in

Editorial supervision: Jill Kramer • *Design:* Tricia Breidenthal
Interior illustration: Mark Hannon

The exercises from *Emergence of the Sensual Woman* by Saida Désilets are used by
permission of the author.

Library of Congress Cataloging-in-Publication Data

Northrup, Christiane.
  The secret pleasures of menopause / Christiane Northrup ; in consultation with
Edward A. Taub, Ferid Murad, and David Oliphant. -- 1st ed.
    p. cm.
  ISBN 978-1-4019-2237-5 (hardcover)
  1. Menopause--Popular works. 2. Middle-aged women--Sexual behavior. 3. Sex
instruction for women. 4. Nitric oxide--Physiological effect. I. Title.
  RG186.N668 2008
  618.1'75--dc22

                                    2008012624

ISBN: 978-1-4019-2237-5

11 10 09 08   4 3 2 1
1st edition, October 2008

Printed in the United States of America

Contents

Introduction

A Brief Overview—
What Is Menopause?

As an obstetrician-gynecologist with more than 30 years of experience on the front lines of women's health, I'm very familiar with everything that can go wrong with the female body. In fact, I've written three books on this topic that have provided women of all ages with a blueprint for changing their perceptions about their bodies as a first step toward better health.

As part of my own midlife rebirth, I've decided to dedicate the second half of my life to teaching women everything that can go *right* with their bodies, including how to experience more pleasure than they've ever dreamed possible. Given our cultural conditioning that we're over the hill at 50 and our best years are behind us, this information is indeed a liberating secret!

The truth is that women over 50 are just hitting their stride. Fifty marks the beginning of the best years of our lives, including the best sex of our lives. As a specialist in women's gynecologic health, I want to get the word out that our bodies were designed to experience unlimited pleasure—and that experiencing this pleasure regularly is part of being vibrantly healthy at any age.

You probably already know what perimenopause and menopause are—and you may be all too familiar with many of the symptoms and physical changes that accompany this life-changing time! But let's briefly review a few main ideas just to reinforce what you already know and also what you can expect.

Menopause (from the Greek words *meno,* meaning "month" or "menses," and *pausis,* meaning "pause") means "the final menstrual period." The average age for women to reach their last period is about 52, but some women go through it as early as 40 and some as late as 58 (give or take a few years). The transitional process leading up to the final menstrual period is called *perimenopause* (from the Greek word *peri,* meaning "around" or "near").

What menopause is *not* is a medical crisis or disorder. Don't worry! Menopause and perimenopause are part of a natural process that involves a gradual change from the ability to conceive and birth a baby to the end of the normal reproductive phase of a woman's life. Since this process lasts on average anywhere from 6 to 13 years, most of us think of it as a stage of life instead of an event. Even so, the official definition of menopause is the point in time when our periods stop permanently. Although most of us were certain of the exact day in adolescence when our periods started, we have no way of knowing when we've had our very last period until an entire year has passed. (Of course, women who've had hysterectomies know the exact date immediately!)

This transition is caused by changes in the brain and body that affect hormone levels, although not all of our hormones decline at the same rate during this time. Estrogen levels actually remain pretty much the same until some time in the final year of the transition, although what does change is the type of estrogen our bodies make. Although they continue to produce some *estradiol,* starting in perimenopause, they shift to making relatively more *estrone* (which is produced both in the ovaries as well as body fat throughout a woman's life, with the exact amount varying a great deal between women).

Although we tend to think of estrogen as the only missing hormone after menopause, the truth is that in many women, progesterone and/or testosterone are often too low as well. Testosterone may or may not decrease; in some women, it actually rises. Progesterone, however, does drop during perimenopause, causing many of the most troublesome symptoms. Progesterone supplementation (with natural, not synthetic progesterone) often helps during early perimenopause when symptoms such as irritability and headaches are primarily related to estrogen dominance. It also helps prevent hot flashes in the latter stages of menopause, probably because progesterone is a precursor hormone that the body can make into estrogen. And it can also relieve angina (chest pain from the heart).

Although for some women, menopausal symptoms are quite bothersome (to say the least), other women seem to sail through the menopausal transition without much of a problem. In either case, the symptoms won't last forever. They're at their height during perimenopause and then taper off and usually disappear altogether within a year or so after the last period.

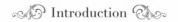

A Range of Symptoms

Here's a rundown of the most common symptoms reported during "the change," although please keep in mind that certainly not all women experience all of them:

— *Irregular periods* are the first sign that the menopausal transition has begun, which typically happens anywhere from two to eight years before a woman's last menstrual period. In fact, women who have previously been as regular as clockwork may go for several months without a period. Even though these irregular periods are a signal that you aren't ovulating every month, that doesn't mean you aren't ovulating *at all*. You may still get pregnant at any time until you reach your one-year mark without a period, so be sure to use birth control if having a baby at this time in your life isn't your intention. Believe me, it happens! Furthermore, pregnancy over the age of 50 increases the risk for both the mother and baby.

— *Lighter or heavier flow during periods* are both common.

— *Hot flashes* are the most common perimeno-pausal symptom, experienced to some degree by up to 85 percent of women. This symptom is at its height near the end of perimenopause. Many women also have night sweats severe enough to wake them, regularly disrupting their sleep. (Night sweats tend to occur between 3 and 4 A.M. for most women, although those who stay up very late at night or who work night shifts may experience a different pattern.)

Hot flashes and night sweats are more severe in women who are under emotional stress, as well as in women who eat a diet high in simple sugars and refined carbohydrates (found in baked goods, candy, white bread, white potatoes, white pasta, wine, liquor, and beer). They are also far more common in women who've had hysterectomies—with or without ovary removal.

— *Mood swings,* such as irritability and depres-sion, are also typical hallmarks of perimenopause. These are especially troublesome for women who previously experienced mood swings before their periods.

— *Insomnia,* even without night sweats, can occur at this time.

— *Fuzzy thinking* (or "cotton head") isn't a sign that dementia is right around the corner, as some women fear, but rather a temporary effect of the hormonal changes of perimenopause. These changes include difficulty concentrating as well as minor forgetfulness. The situation is similar to the mental fuzziness many women experience after giving birth. "Cotton head" is designed to turn your attention inward so that you can focus on yourself for a change!

— *Heart palpitations* during the menopausal transition are experienced by women with higher levels of stress hormones caused by, among other things, greater levels of fear and anxiety. Often, this arises from past trauma that you now have the strength to resolve once and for all. (Heart palpitations can also be a sign of thyroid imbalance.) Chest pain (angina) can also occur and is related both to stress hormones and lack of progesterone.

— *Migraines* may occur more often in perimenopause, usually (but not always) in women who previously experienced migraines in the days before their period. These are often triggered by falling progesterone levels.

— *Breast tenderness* can also occur more frequently in women who previously experienced it premenstrually. (Breast tenderness is often a sign of iodine deficiency, too.)

— *Bone loss* can be a problem, especially for women who don't eat a healthy diet and don't exercise. (Bone loss is also a sign of vitamin D deficiency.) All women should have their vitamin D levels checked.

— *Hypothyroidism* that often has no overt symptoms and can only be diagnosed with proper testing occurs in up to one quarter of women at this time. In many women, this is caused by iodine deficiency. To test whether you may have it, just paint a patch of ammonium iodide (known as Iosol) on your wrist in the morning (it's available at **www.TPCSdirect.com**). (In dark-skinned women, put it on an area where skin is lightest.) It should still be visible when you go to bed at night, 10 to 12 hours later. If the iodine "disappears" earlier than that, you may need more iodine in your diet. You can get it by eating sea vegetables and seafood or by taking Iosol regularly—one to two drops a day or as directed by your health-care provider. Another great source is Modifilan (**www.modifilan.com**), a concentrated organic seaweed extract. Recheck your iodine absorption every six weeks or so thereafter. *Note:* Replenishing iodine levels can lower the need for thyroid hormones, so be sure to monitor your thyroid hormone levels.

— *Benign uterine fibroids* (noncancerous tumors made up of muscle and connective tissue) develop in about 40 percent of women.

— *Changes in sex drive* are also common. Contrary to popular belief, the hormone changes during menopause don't lower sex drive in healthy women. For some women, however, a drop in testosterone from drugs, surgery, or adrenal exhaustion can reduce sexual desire. Changes in estrogen levels also reduce sex drive in some, in addition to causing vaginal dryness and irritation that make intercourse painful. (By the way, this can be easily alleviated with lubricants or topical estrogen creams available by prescription.) For women who've reached the one-year mark without a period, however, the freedom from the worry of unwanted pregnancy can actually be one factor in *heightening* sex drive.

Brain chemistry also changes in midlife, affecting the way we think and process information. For example, midlife women often find that they not only have stronger feelings about injustice and unfairness, but they're also more willing to speak up about them. Because the temporal lobes in the brain are more often engaged, our intuition is enhanced. But unlike most of the symptoms in the previous list, the shifts in our brain chemistry are more or less permanent—a sign that we really do get wiser as life progresses.

You may also find that you have a much stronger creative drive now since your life energy isn't being used in order to have periods and create babies. Instead, it gets rerouted into powerful urges to create other things—anything from a personal journal of poetry and sketches to a thriving new business. Long-buried dreams and feelings resurface with a renewed passion at this time. It's as if your soul is saying, *Hey— what about me? When is it my turn?* If you don't act on your innermost dreams and desires now and instead hold them in—usually out of fear of disrupting or upsetting family members—then you're apt to have a much harder time with menopausal symptoms. But that's not all. You'll also be setting yourself up for health problems down the road.

The bottom line is that we women are designed to be more in touch with what really matters to us after menopause, and our bodies act as incredibly accurate barometers that indicate how closely we live our lives in-line with our true heart's desires. When we get out of line with what we really want, we get a gentle nudge to warn us to make changes that will put us back on course. If we don't pay attention, the nudge may turn into a shove!

When you look at menopause from this perspective, you'll realize that your midlife body is Divinely designed to help you make choices that will keep you healthy and happy. Now what could be better than that?

Suffering Isn't Inevitable

How distressing your physical and emotional symptoms are during perimenopause depends on how out of balance with wellness your lifestyle has been in the years leading up to this point. Think of it this way: Your body has given you about 40 years or so to get your act together. During your teens, 20s, and 30s, your body is incredibly forgiving. If you're overstressed, overworked, or drink too much; if you smoke, underexercise, and eat a poor diet, you may still be able to maintain moderately good health.

But once you reach midlife, your body will no longer let you get away with this kind of lifestyle, and you'll eventually pay the price. So why not make changes for the better now! Women who approach menopause in a state of emotional and nutritional depletion typically have the most serious perimenopausal symptoms—not to mention poorer health as they age. On the other hand, studies show that women who have been eating right, exercising regularly, and taking good care of themselves don't tend to suffer from bone loss, low sex drive, cardiovascular problems, depression, forgetfulness, or other common menopausal challenges. Good news, right?

Your mind is also a key part in how easily you make this transition. Your attitudes, thoughts, beliefs, and expectations greatly impact how you experience menopause. Let me tell you about the women in the !Kung tribe in southern Africa. These women enjoy a higher social status after menopause, and as a result, instead of dreading the transition, they very much look forward to it. Their entire culture is in agreement with this belief. Not surprisingly, the !Kung don't have menopausal symptoms; in fact, they don't even have a word for "hot flash" in their language!

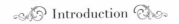

The Change—in How We Look at Midlife

The common belief in society has long been that menopause means you're getting old, and that's why your body is meant to start falling apart. But in reality, nothing could be further from the truth. You're just experiencing what I call "breakdown to breakthrough." The best is yet to come!

The menopausal transition is a wake-up call that's urging you to make changes that will keep you in touch with your vital life force (sometimes called *chi* or *prana*). The truth about this time of life is that when you have the courage to change your beliefs and behaviors so that you speak your truth and dare to cultivate pleasure instead of stress, you have the power to create a life of unbridled joy, unlimited abundance, and vibrant health. That absolutely includes having the best sex of your life . . . now that's something to look forward to!

CHAPTER ONE

It's Not Over!

The end of our childbearing years may be the end of one season, but it certainly doesn't mean that it's all over and we're washed up—far from it! Even though this has been the conventional view for decades, the only thing that truly ends at menopause is a woman's ability to naturally conceive a child. (I use the word *naturally* because thanks to the latest scientific developments, postmenopausal women can—with a little help from technology— get pregnant and even give birth!) Instead of being an ending, menopause is really the beginning of our coming into our power in a whole new way. It's the springtime of the second half of life, and what many women are finding is that it's the *best* half of life!

Even though menopause isn't the end, it can certainly feel like it sometimes. The reason is simple—throughout much of human history, menopause *did* represent the end for many women. At the beginning of the 20th century, the average life expectancy for women was only 40 years.

The other reason why menopause can seem like the end is because this is a time when many of us feel the need to let go of whatever isn't working in our lives. This includes jobs, relationships, and lifestyles that don't support the fullness of who we're becoming. Letting go of our past requires faith and is rarely easy. But in the words of author Joseph Campbell, "We must be willing to get rid of the life we've planned, so as to have the life that is waiting for us."

And there's a *lot* of life that is waiting for us after menopause. The average life expectancy for women today is well over 80! Not only are we living longer, but we're also living healthier than ever before. Cancer rates have gone down since 1991, and the number of women dying of heart disease has decreased five years in a row for the first time in written history. If a woman today reaches her 50th birthday without having had cancer or heart disease, she can expect to still be kicking at 92. The way this trend is going, someday women may live more years after menopause than they will before it!

We also no longer need to fear becoming mentally feeble in our later years. A study presented at the 2006 gathering of the Society for Neuroscience showed that with the right training, the brain of an 85-year-old can work just as adeptly as that of a 30-year-old. Good news!

The bottom line is that physical and mental decline is *not* a natural consequence of aging, as we've been led to believe. It's largely a consequence of our culture's *beliefs* about aging and of our lifestyle choices. However, those beliefs are changing rapidly as baby-boomer women reach midlife in record-breaking numbers. According to estimates by the U.S. Census Bureau, one in five adults in the U.S. today is a woman over 50.

Take a good look around and you'll see what I mean: Older women have never been emotionally stronger, economically more powerful, or physically more sexy and beautiful than they are right now!

Even better, fewer of us need convincing. Almost six out of ten women between the ages 50 and 70 like what they see when they look in the mirror, according to research reported by Marti Barletta in *PrimeTime Women*. Not only that, but a whopping 82 percent of women in this age group feel a lot younger than their actual age, and 59 percent believe their greatest achievements are still ahead of them. Clearly, the image of the menopausal woman as a dried-up has-been no longer holds true.

I need look no further than my 82-year-old mother, Edna, for proof. In her late 60s, she hiked the entire Appalachian Trail. At 70, she spent three months hiking and kayaking in Alaska. Several years later, she climbed the 200 highest peaks in New England with her friend Anne, who is three years older than she is. And a few years ago, she climbed Mount Washington and went snowshoeing in northern Vermont with a 90-year-old friend. I'm beginning to wonder if she's even hit middle age yet!

Giving Birth Again

The physical and emotional discomfort many of us experience at perimenopause is in effect the labor pains of giving birth to our new, best selves. Instead of using our energy for everyone and everything else around us, as we did when we were raising our families and nurturing our careers, we're now biologically called to focus that energy on ourselves.

If you can't imagine putting yourself first, look at it this way: There's a reason why flight attendants instruct those who are traveling with small children to put the oxygen mask on themselves *first* in the event that they drop from the overhead compartments. You can't help *anyone* if you don't take care of yourself first—if you don't, *everyone* loses.

For women who have reveled in the challenge, satisfaction, and even admiration of being the center of their families, giving up that position can be difficult indeed. It helps to realize that by updating our roles and giving up some of the reins of family control, we'll be setting a good example for our grown children. How fabulous to present our daughters (or daughters-in-law, grandchildren, or nieces) with a midlife role model whose life includes freedom, fulfillment, and fun as opposed to being stuck in duty and drudgery.

Would you want your children to hold back who they're fully capable of becoming? Of course not! Neither should you.

Rebirthing ourselves may involve rocking the boat a bit. It may call for disrupting the status quo, bucking convention, and saying no when we might otherwise have said yes (or vice versa). A big part of this transition is letting go of what we've outgrown that no longer serves us—the roles and relationships that hold us back and take more energy from us than they give us.

Here's an example from my own life: I bought a Mustang convertible to enjoy for myself, but on nice days, my daughter wanted to use it, too. So I let her. As a mother, I enjoy making her happy, but always giving in meant that I never had a chance to drive around with the top down myself! I realized that by doing this, I was engaging in what amounted to unhealthy self-sacrifice. So I soon started driving my convertible whenever I wanted to, and it felt great!

Whatever doesn't feed our soul and doesn't make us feel vibrantly alive needs to fall by the wayside now. Our lives have no room for such things anymore. Everything we think, say, and do from this point on will either keep us actively engaged in living passionately and joyfully, or it will hasten degeneration and increase our chances of poor health and disease. It's our choice to make.

Know also that this emotional housecleaning isn't a onetime event. It becomes a new way of life. As soon as you recognize that something isn't working for you anymore, you always have the opportunity to make a new choice that fits your needs better.

The Cleansing Fire of Anger

Stormy emotions typically accompany the midlife transition. One of the emotions that often fuels this personal rebirth is anger. Anger is a sign that you've been putting up with things that haven't served you fully—and you're not willing to put up with them anymore. The anger of midlife women is the brunt of many jokes. But believe me, this anger is like jet fuel—it's the energy needed to propel you into your new life.

One of the reasons why anger surfaces is because we feel an almost fierce need to have our say and to be heard—sometimes for the first time in decades. Many of us stifled our true voice sometime in adolescence, when we were more concerned with fitting in, finding our place, and following the rules. Now that we're redefining who we are, we can no longer put a lid on what upsets us, and with good reason. Although we may be used to thinking of anger as a negative, in the midlife transition it can be seen as a measure of the strength of our vital life force. In fact, if the symptoms of perimenopause are the labor pains we experience as we give birth to our authentic selves at midlife, then our anger is the cry of our newborn selves whom we've just birthed.

The Power of Midlife Passion

Passion is another emotion we often unleash with renewed intensity at this time of life. Many midlife women feel a growing enthusiasm for activities they previously put on the back burner and report that their lives change for the better when they start engaging in pursuits that excite them. Such activities can include things like reading books, going to the movies with friends, traveling, horseback riding, creating artwork, being out in nature, writing poetry, and even redecorating (in other words, anything enjoyable that they never took the time to do). This can also include volunteering for a cause that's greater than themselves. There's something life-giving and life-enhancing about lending our efforts toward the greater good. And believe it or not, the good feelings that come from giving back can also spill over into our sex lives!

Indulging in our passions is an important part of our midlife passage because it helps us connect at a deep emotional and spiritual level with our newly emerging selves. These activities aren't a luxury. Doing what we love and what brings us pleasure keeps our life force well stoked. This is definitely a time to, as the saying goes, follow our bliss.

There's something vitally important that you should know about what happens when you do this: Women who make a point of maintaining a strong, passionate life force become magnetically attractive to uplifting people and circumstances. (Statistics show that they also add about eight years to their lives!) So while you're having a great time with all of the wonderful things you're bringing into your life, you'll also be sending out signals that say to the universe, *I'm loving life and loving that I love life, so bring on more of the good stuff!* The universe always responds, because whatever you give your attention to grows. And when you give your attention to bringing life-affirming, fun things into your life, you open up a channel for more of the same to come in. It's as simple as that.

In fact, this feeling of being in love with life itself is absolutely vital if you want to have a passionate, fulfilling relationship with a partner. After all, you can't give what you don't have. Ratcheting up the passion, excitement, and enthusiasm in all areas of your life will also help you increase the passion in your current relationship or help you attract a mate with whom you can have a red-hot relationship. In other words, before you can have a passionate relationship with someone else, you have to already be in a passionate relationship—with yourself and your life.

Here's why passion is a vital key in your life. When you allow joy and pleasure into your life, you're more in touch with your truest self, and that's the self who will be attracting others to you. That authentic self is powerful, beautiful, and positively intoxicating to others who likewise have the same level of passion in their lives. (And believe it or not, your true essence is much more attractive than the person you think you should be or the person you want everyone to think you are!) So the way it works is that as these other people who are in love with life are sending out their upbeat signals, you'll be able to pick up on them as surely and easily as they're picking up on yours. Like attracts like. It's one of the laws of the universe!

I want to stress that there is no age limit for having a passionate relationship of any kind—including having a passionate sex life. Although society often leads us to believe that menopause means the death of sexual desire, that kind of thinking is definitely outmoded. As long as we maintain vibrant physical and emotional health, we can maintain a vibrantly healthy sex life. Going through menopause doesn't decrease sexual desire in women who are healthy and happy. In fact, the number one predictor of a strong libido at menopause is having a new sexual partner—even for women who previously had less-than-wonderful sex lives.

This doesn't mean you should dump your partner. It means that you yourself can *become* a new partner. As long as your head and heart are willing, your body will find a way.

Another important key to a healthy sex life, no matter how old you are, is that any woman can learn to turn her body on. It's true! But doing so isn't something you can address only in bed. Sexual desire starts with an idea and is fueled by your thoughts and attitudes as much as it is by any physical action or response. You don't need to have the body of a young woman to be sexy and desirable. You simply have to start thinking of yourself as a sexually desirable woman! As human sexuality researcher Gina Ogden, Ph.D., puts it, "Self-esteem is the mother of sexual desire, and that desire can ripen with age—like fine wine."

When you have the courage to go through the cleansing fires of perimenopause, you emerge from the other side into the life that is, indeed, waiting for you.

And you find that it's better than you ever dreamed it could be!

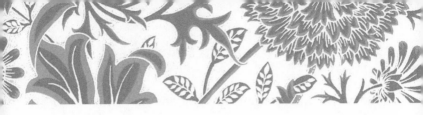

·✧· CHAPTER TWO ·✧·

Experience
Unlimited Pleasure

We humans were born to experience unlimited pleasure and joy. It's our birthright. Pursuing pleasure and also allowing ourselves to receive it on a regular basis are absolutely essential to creating and maintaining vibrant physical and emotional health. That's right—the pursuit of good feelings is *not* an indulgence. It's a life-affirming necessity! Pleasure in all its many forms literally stokes our life force (our *chi* or *prana*) in the way we'd stoke a fire by throwing another log onto it.

Think about the last time you really steeped yourself in something pleasurable—when you took that positive feeling right into your bone marrow.

Maybe it was savoring a bite of gourmet chocolate, the smell of salt air at the beach, or an exquisite back rub. Everyone has a distinct pleasure profile, and you can count on your senses to let you know when you've dialed into yours. Remember the intensity of your pleasure. (If you can't remember what it feels like to lose yourself in bliss, hang around a two-year-old for five minutes.) When you're lost in the joy of pleasure, you are, in that very moment, renewing your cells, increasing your blood circulation, and creating health on all levels—body, mind, and spirit. In fact, you're probably getting a healthful boost right now just imagining that wonderful experience all over again!

Another way to understand how potent pleasure is as a health enhancer is to imagine what happens when you aren't feeling any of it. Think about a time when you were totally burned out. You probably felt like you were running on empty, right? Guess what? You were! It wasn't just energy you were lacking; it was vital life force. Compare them in this way: Energy is what it takes to get through the day. Vital life force is what it takes to put spring in your step as you get through the day. See the difference?

Because pleasure fuels your life force, you're naturally drawn to it by Divine design. Your body

14

is actually programmed for joy! But before I go any further, let me explain what pleasure is *not*. Pleasure isn't getting drunk or high and doing things that will embarrass you the next day; and it doesn't mean renouncing your family and job to go live in a spa or escape to a desert island. Even though cutting loose once in a while can provide you with a temporary high that relieves tension, getting high, drunk, or going on a sugar binge won't provide you with sustained pleasure—or vibrant health. Most likely, you'll end up feeling worse. Avoiding responsibility and being physically, emotionally, or even financially reckless actually undermines your ability to maintain positive feelings.

When I recommend the pursuit of pleasure, I'm talking about learning how to recognize and value the things that bring you lasting joy, and then bringing them into your life deliberately on a regular basis. Think of it this way: Your body itself was conceived in orgasm—the most exquisite pleasure humans are capable of experiencing. From that perspective, how could pleasure *not* play a vital role in the optimal functioning of your body?

Why Pleasure and Health Are Related

Just as any piece of machinery works better when it's properly lubricated, your organs (and the rest of your body) work better when you're thinking thoughts and feeling emotions that bring you pleasure or when you're pursuing enjoyable activities. That's true in several ways.

First of all, experiencing pleasure improves blood flow. Healthy blood flow is important because the bloodstream brings nutrients to all of your body's cells and carries away the cells' waste products. It's like stocking the fridge and emptying the garbage at the same time.

All of this happens by virtue of a gas called *nitric oxide*. When you're experiencing pleasure or feeling calm, vibrant, and healthy, nitric oxide is released in little puffs mostly from the lining of your blood vessels. Because it's a gas, it diffuses rapidly in all directions—right through cell walls. It's equivalent to e-mail blasts occurring almost instantly all over your body. Not only does this result in increased circulation, but nitric oxide also turns on the production of special chemicals in your body called *neurotransmitters*. Neurotransmitters carry myriad messages between the brain and nervous system, helping your body work and feel better.

One of the neurotransmitters that pleasure increases is called *beta-endorphin,* which acts sort of like morphine—it dulls pain and creates feelings of euphoria. This not only improves your mood, but it also helps you deal more effectively with the stresses of life. Another neurotransmitter that pleasure boosts is called *prolactin* (which is also known as the hormone of bonding). Prolactin is released when you nurse a child, have an orgasm, or even get together with good friends. It makes you feel bonded to the person (or people) you're interacting with at the time. Prolactin supports loving feelings between mothers and their infants, women and their mates, and even between friends.

Speaking of orgasm and sex, perhaps the most obvious proof that our bodies were designed for pleasure is the existence of the clitoris. This fleshy little budlike organ, which is connected to deeper erectile tissue in the pelvis, sits right above the vaginal opening, partially covered and protected by a hood of skin. Despite its small external size (it's no bigger than a pencil eraser), it contains 8,000 nerve endings that increase sexual excitement and ultimately bring on orgasm.

Although some people mistakenly assume that women urinate through this organ, thinking it does double duty like a man's penis, this isn't the case. Instead, women urinate from a tiny hole located between the clitoris and the vagina. The clitoris has nothing to do with urinating—or even with conception or reproduction. It's actually the only organ in the human body whose sole purpose is pleasure. (Talk about being hardwired for good times!)

Every time you feel pleasure in your clitoral area, you're also flooding yourself in nitric oxide, which, as we've just seen, radically improves the health of your whole body. We'll talk *much* more about the life-enhancing effects of nitric oxide in the next chapter, including how you can increase the levels of this miraculous molecule in your body. But for now, just know that this is yet another way that pleasure enhances your health on many levels and in many ways!

If you've ever read my other books or heard me speak, you know that I talk a lot about the fact that your body has wisdom to share with you. If you listen to the language of your body through the various physical symptoms you experience, you'll be better able to understand your heart's true desire and create vibrant health both physically and emotionally.

Well, ladies, the truth is that our orgasms have wisdom to share with us, too! Female orgasms are, in fact, a metaphor, illustrating how pleasure works both in our bodies and in our lives.

Let me explain what I mean by that. To begin with, you can't experience orgasm when you're tense and upset. And it's not even enough just to be relaxed. To climax, nothing less than total surrender to pleasure is required. You must give yourself over fully to the sensation of pleasure, or the bell doesn't ring. It's as simple as that!

This requires getting out of your head and into your body. You can't force yourself to have an orgasm by willing it with your mind, but when the frontal lobes in the brain are turned off during sleep, it's not only possible, it's also normal to reach climaxes while dreaming. This is proof that your body knows how to receive such pleasure! You just have to learn to allow those 8,000 clitoral nerve endings (and the other pleasure circuits in the body that are connected to them, such as the G-spot or "sacred" spot just behind the pubic bone on the top of the vagina) to do their job so that you can experience as much pleasure as possible. There's no ceiling on sensual delight. You can even learn how to become multiorgasmic!

It's the same way with cultivating joy in your life. If you really desire the rejuvenating magic of pleasure, you have to open up to it, trust it, and allow it to flood your being. The journey starts by simply noticing and enjoying the sensation of a gentle breeze on your skin!

Because women often need time to become sexually aroused and climax, some feel like there's a flaw in the system or that the design doesn't work quite right. *But exactly the opposite is true.* What your body in its infinite wisdom is trying to tell you is that it's okay to take your time! Your body was designed to take the slow route, not the fast-track shortcut. You deserve all the love and attention that it takes for you to get there. In fact, the key to experiencing more orgasmic pleasure is, ironically, learning to enjoy every stroke and sensation along the way without even thinking about the "goal" of orgasm. You reach your optimal peak of both pleasure and health not through the quick fix, but through a long-term, sustained attention to cultivating pleasure. This is as true in life as it is between the sheets.

Why We Push Pleasure Away

But this isn't the message we've been getting from society, is it? Unfortunately, most of us are used to thinking of pleasure as a dessert we can eat only if we have the time, money, and room for it, instead of as one of the major food groups. The majority of us don't make pursuing pleasure a priority in our lives because our pleasure-starved culture talks us out of it. We say that we don't have the time and that other things are far more important. We're made to feel guilty for even *thinking* about doing something solely for our own pleasure. (Where do you think the expression "guilty pleasure" came from?)

Our culture (or sometimes our family) definitely gives people bonus points for pain and suffering. In fact, many individuals try to outdo each other in this regard. ("That's nothing," someone says after listening to a hair-raising tale. "Listen to what happened to me!") After all, we're living in a society where one of the major mottos is "No pain, no gain."

Society teaches the belief that there's a lot of value in blood, sweat, and tears; and suffering and playing the martyr are holy. That's half right. Hard work and effort can indeed be good for anyone. When you push yourself to be all you can be, going past what you thought were your limits, you benefit enormously. But suffering has never been a necessary part of the equation. Making it a way of life or wearing it like a badge of honor does nothing but attract more misery to you. And being a martyr never made anyone a better person (except maybe Joan of Arc, and look what happened to *her!*).

The key is balance. Too much of *anything* isn't good for you, and that includes hard work and effort. When you work too hard, push yourself too far, and allow yourself to become stressed over everything you think you *have* to do rather than giving serious consideration to what your heart is *longing* to do, you're doing yourself a grave disservice. When this imbalance continues long enough, the results are often disastrous to your well-being.

The effect of denying yourself pleasure or pushing it away is sort of like what happens when you hold your breath. At first it feels uncomfortable, and then it gets downright unpleasant as your body screams for what it needs. You can easily imagine what would happen if you denied your body air. But what you might not realize is that by denying yourself pleasure, you're doing something that is similarly damaging.

Damage Report

Here's how the damage happens: When you lead a stressful lifestyle and don't concentrate on bringing pleasure into your life on a regular basis, your body makes stress hormones that restrict blood flow and your nitric oxide levels plummet. As a result, so do your levels of the neurotransmitter beta-endorphin (that's the one that's like morphine). You're likely to feel sad, depressed, and maybe even edgy or angry. You get irritated easily. And chances are, you reach for something to make you feel better.

Often what you reach for is a quick ecstasy fix through sugary junk food, alcohol, coffee, cigarettes, or drugs. You might even tell yourself that because of how hard you're working or how much stress you're under, you deserve this little treat. And because you really do feel better momentarily after you eat the doughnut or drink the wine, you convince yourself that it really does help. But what's really happening when you indulge in overeating, smoking, drinking to get drunk, or taking drugs to get high (or even such practices as sadomasochistic sex) is that you're numbing yourself so that you don't have to feel any of your unpleasant, or even downright painful, feelings. And the more you turn to those quick fixes, the more numb you become over time.

That kind of "help" backfires in the long run because your body gets used to your mood-altering substances of choice. And then you need more in order to achieve the same effect. It becomes a vicious cycle—not the best route to optimal health! In fact, that's how addiction and disease get started. Pursuing pleasure and allowing yourself to receive it in your day-to-day life, on the other hand, produces significantly better and more long-lasting results.

Saying Yes to Pleasure

So how do you invite joy and pleasure into your everyday life? By bathing your brain and body in a constant supply of nitric oxide! And there are many ways to do this that don't involve drugs, alcohol, or sugar. These include anything that gives you sustainable pleasure and creates vibrant health in your body. In addition to following your bliss, the list includes exercise, meditation, and orgasm. (At the moment of orgasm, there's a blast of life-giving nitric oxide—which also bumps up levels of all the other feel-good neurotransmitters.)

Regularly engaging in any or all of these activities keeps your nitric oxide levels high. But the trick is the word *regular*. It's like putting money in your retirement account: If you only make a deposit once in a while, it won't really do much for you, but if you're disciplined enough to make annual contributions, you'll be surprised and pleased by how much your money has grown! So that's the good news: Pleasure (including sex and specifically orgasm) isn't just a good time. It's part of the way your body resets its electromagnetic grid to maintain vibrant health and well-being.

Ready to get started? Since your body was designed for pleasure, the steps for experiencing more of it are pretty straightforward:

1. Desire it! You must put aside any remaining feelings of guilt you may have about the pursuit of pleasure. Hopefully by now, you've come to see pleasure as a health-affirming necessity rather than a sin to resist.

2. Know you deserve it! Even if you believe that we as humans are programmed to seek out pleasure, you must understand that you, personally, deserve it. Pleasure and joy aren't just for everyone else—they're for you, too. You were born with a clitoris, after all. Case closed!

3. Believe! Yes, you *can* learn to bring more pleasure into your life on a daily basis. And yes, your body *will* respond to that pleasure with optimal health.

4. Overcome your resistance! Whenever your doubts start to creep in, simply notice them. Then choose pleasure anyway. It may be difficult to reprogram yourself to think of feeling joy as your birthright instead of as a sinful luxury, but the more you do so, the easier it will become. You'll soon see and feel the results—including more sparkle in your eyes, glowing skin, and a springier step!

5. Learn to receive pleasure and embrace it! If someone offered you a hundred one-dollar bills with absolutely no strings attached and also told you that there was an unlimited supply of them being offered to everyone, would you take just a few dollars and walk away? That may sound like a far-fetched scenario, but it's what happens when you give in halfheartedly to your desires—you get only a little joy and a little benefit back.

All the fullness of your passion and delight is just waiting for you to claim it. And when you do, it will change your world for the better—guaranteed. What are you waiting for?

CHAPTER THREE

Discover the Nitric Oxide Pleasure Connection

To experience the maximal amount of pleasure possible (not to mention the greatest sex you've ever had at midlife and beyond), you must follow a lifestyle that enhances the production of an amazing molecule called nitric oxide (NO). This simple molecule is made of one atom of nitrogen and one atom of oxygen. When it's produced in the environment by car engines and power plants, nitric oxide is a toxic air pollutant. But don't let that scare you, because the nitric oxide that's made inside your body is extremely beneficial.

Nitric oxide is a free radical, which is normally something doctors advise patients to guard against because most free radicals attack cells and cause damage. But just as there is good cholesterol (HDL) and bad cholesterol (LDL), medical researchers have discovered that there are good and bad free radicals as well. (By the way, don't confuse nitric oxide with *nitrous* oxide, an anesthetic some dentists use that's commonly known as laughing gas.)

Nitric oxide is special because, quite simply, it resets your power grid and reboots your body the same way you reboot your computer in order to make it work better. The more nitric oxide your body makes on a regular basis, the healthier and happier you are on many levels. Nitric oxide is the mother of all "feel good" molecules; and it isn't illegal, immoral, or the least bit fattening! In fact, it's quite the reverse. It's perfectly natural, it's easy (and fun) to increase once you know how, and it's the key to developing and maintaining optimum health. Think of it as your secret weapon for wellness!

One of my partners and a medical consultant for this book, Ferid Murad, M.D., Ph.D., shared the 1998 Nobel Prize in Medicine for his research leading to the discovery that nitric oxide is the body's signaling molecule. This means that if your body makes enough nitric oxide, your cells stay healthy and function well, but if your levels aren't high enough, then your cells begin to break down. And this sets the stage for aches, pains, and the kind of chronic degenerative diseases that are associated with aging, such as diabetes, heart disease, cancer, and arthritis. Let me explain how this book came about.

Dr. Murad wrote a book entitled *The Wellness Solution* with Edward A. Taub, M.D., a wellness pioneer; and David Oliphant, a former minor-league pitcher for the New York Yankees and the Los Angeles Dodgers who went on to become a successful publishing icon. Their collaboration led to the mind-boggling conclusion that nitric oxide is the spark of life! I had already written about the importance of nitric oxide in my previous books, but their bold vision led me to see it in a whole new light. It's the actual molecule that determines physical, emotional, spiritual, and sexual wellness in menopausal women (and everyone else). Wow!

We discussed applying my nitric oxide insight to writing a much-needed book with explicit advice about better sex and more pleasure after menopause—all backed up by Nobel Prize–winning science. Since then, we've all become partners, and I consult with them in their special areas of expertise.

What Nitric Oxide Is and How It Works Its Magic

Nitric oxide is an invisible, odorless gas that your body makes, mostly in the lining of your blood vessels in the endothelium, an extremely thin but very important layer. Other areas in your body produce nitric oxide as well, including lung cells, white blood cells, and neurons (the nerve cells in the brain).

When nitric oxide is produced, it causes the smooth muscles in the walls of your blood vessels to relax. (That's right—even your blood vessels have muscles!) When those muscles are relaxed, the blood vessels open or widen, allowing more life-supporting oxygen and other nutrients to get to your heart, brain, and all of your other organs. With enough nitric oxide, the circulation throughout your entire body improves. The effect is the same as adding a few extra lanes to a highway during rush hour—instead of the usual traffic jams, everything moves more quickly and smoothly, and everyone is much happier as a result!

Some drugs rely on nitric oxide as well. For example, the prescription drug nitroglycerin releases nitric oxide, increasing blood flow to the heart that, in turn, eases chest pain in patients with angina. The

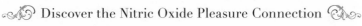

same principle is at work with drugs such as Viagra, which helps men achieve and keep erections. With this class of drugs, nitric oxide is released from nerve cells in the blood vessels of the penis. This relaxes the blood vessels, allowing more blood flow and therefore improved erections. But fortunately, nitric oxide does a whole lot more than ease chest pain and enable erections, and because the body produces it naturally, you don't need to take it as a drug to benefit!

You might imagine that wider blood vessels and improved circulation would reduce high blood pressure, and you're right. But that's not all. We now know that all diseases—including the big killers such as heart disease, stroke, cancer, and diabetes—are associated with cellular inflammation, which restricts blood flow by lowering nitric oxide levels. On the other hand, anything that keeps your blood vessels soft, elastic, and open also helps prevent cellular inflammation and all the various chronic degenerative diseases associated with it. The end result is a healthy, youthful body. Pretty impressive!

There's more, too. Because nitric oxide is a gas, it can pass right through your cell membranes, not at all restricted by cell walls. This is important because the nitric oxide that's made in the neurons in your brain actually acts as a special kind of neurotransmitter, easily and instantly sending messages from one part of your brain to another. This includes the "thinking" parts (those used for conscious thought, such as deciding to pick something up or walk across the room) and the "nonthinking" parts (those that regulate the autonomic nervous system, which control heart rate, blood pressure, breathing, and everything else that the body does without your having to think about it).

That's pretty significant (as I'll discuss later in this chapter), because your conscious "thinking" brain is always talking to the "nonthinking" parts of your brain that control your bodily functions. It's just that you're not consciously aware of the powerful effect that your conscious brain (and thoughts) have on the nonthinking parts of your brain that control your health! It turns out that nitric oxide is the molecule that makes that connection—instantly. When you have the thought, *I'm completely capable of and willing to change for the better!* this powerfully healthy sentiment spontaneously sends increased nitric oxide levels to every organ of your body!

Nitric oxide not only sends messages from your brain to every part of your body in order to help sustain optimal health in everything from your heart and lungs to your bones and muscles, it also sends signals that allow your body to maintain health by solving problems. For example, it can signal white blood cells to fight infection and kill tumors, it can initiate the repair of damaged tissue, and it can even reduce the stickiness of blood clots that can lead to heart attacks and strokes. Not only that, nitric oxide also transmits messages from all over your body back to your brain, letting your brain know that its initial messages have been received and acted upon.

There are other neurotransmitters in the brain besides nitric oxide that travel to all parts of the body, of course, but here's the advantage that nitric oxide has: Because it's a gas, the nitric oxide molecules diffuse rapidly in all directions at the same time, instead of affecting only the neurons near them as they pass the information. In other words, nitric oxide sends its messages of health and well-being almost instantaneously throughout your entire brain and body. It's the difference between using a state-of-the-art sound system to communicate with an entire crowd, including those in the very back, and playing "whisper down the lane," hoping that each person will repeat the message clearly and effectively without garbling it in the process. It's not hard to figure out which way you'd rather get an important message across, is it?

Nitric oxide even works its magic at the very start of life. Research done on sea urchins at Stanford University shows that when sperm and egg are united, nitric oxide is immediately manufactured and released in first the sperm and then the egg. It's this discharge of nitric oxide that triggers the vital release of calcium that's necessary for the newly fertilized egg to start the process of dividing and becoming an embryo. Researchers believe that this process probably works much the same for humans as well.

The latest findings also indicate that providing nitric oxide to the lungs of premature babies can save their lives. (Interestingly, the white light that so many people report as part of near-death experiences is also from a blast of nitric oxide—leading me to believe that the energy that gets us into our physical bodies is present when we exit as well. This thought can really help us trust the process of life.)

Nitric oxide is, quite literally, the spark of life— the physical equivalent of life energy, *chi,* or *prana.* It's what breathes life into us in the first place, and then throughout our lives, it tells our cells to live or die, to thrive or decay. If we can learn to raise our levels of nitric oxide naturally and regularly, we can truly experience vibrant health every day of our lives. Who wouldn't want that? I know I certainly do!

Getting Enough Nitric Oxide

So how do we increase and maintain our levels of this miraculous molecule? That's a very important question, because the truth is that most Americans just don't have enough nitric oxide in their bodies—especially as they get older. Factors like obesity, lack of exercise, poor nutrition, smoking, and high levels of stress all decrease our levels of nitric oxide. And that, in turn, makes us more vulnerable to disease and poor health.

The good news is that no matter how low your nitric oxide levels are right now, you can take action to boost them significantly. The first step is living a healthy lifestyle that includes choosing uplifting thoughts and telling positive stories about yourself, such as: *Every day is full of joyous opportunities.* This is the exact opposite of assuming the "victim role." It's essential to be in touch with and learn how to healthfully express all of your emotions—including grief, fear, and anger. So when you're angry, feel it and express it (safely). Next, take a moment to discover why you feel that way, and then take steps to change your response to the situation. In addition, take active steps to change the situation itself whenever possible.

Assuming this empowered stance in life is the first step that automatically leads to sustainable changes in your lifestyle, including eating nutritious foods, maintaining a healthy weight, drinking enough water, taking the right kind of supplements (high in antioxidants), stopping smoking, getting sufficient sleep, reducing stress, and increasing pleasure. I'll go into each of these areas in much more detail in the following chapters, but for now, it's enough to know that you can take charge of your health and turn it around no matter where your starting point is. So take heart!

Depending on your current state of health, you may also need to work with a health-care professional to control conditions such as high cholesterol and a poor lipid profile, high blood pressure, and diabetes—all of which can contribute to low levels of nitric oxide in your body. Please note that there are many good natural alternatives to drugs for these conditions; however, prescription drugs may sometimes be necessary.

As you learn the process of increasing your levels of nitric oxide naturally, keep this in mind: Creating optimal nitric oxide levels requires a true commitment to changing your life. Nitric oxide can't be socked away like money in the bank and then

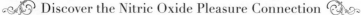

taken out in chunks when you need it. The lifespan of this incredible molecule is only a few seconds! It's produced as it's needed, on the spot—if the conditions are right. So to achieve and maintain optimal health, you have to keep your body producing nitric oxide on a regular basis. It's a renewable resource because your body is capable of manufacturing an ever-abundant supply—but that doesn't happen automatically. You must learn to cultivate it. And remember, because a *big* part of optimizing nitric oxide production involves focusing more on bringing pleasure into your life, it's not as daunting a suggestion as you might otherwise think!

The Mind-Body Connection and Nitric Oxide

Reducing stress is important in raising nitric oxide levels because negative emotions such as anger, hurt, disappointment, fear, and worry all deplete nitric oxide. In fact, researchers suspect that it's a vicious cycle and that insufficient levels of nitric oxide may trigger negative emotions as well. So learning how to get off of that downward spiral is essential to optimal health.

The reverse is also true: Increasing your pleasure (which begins with thinking pleasurable and positive thoughts) increases nitric oxide throughout your body. Activities like yoga, massage, acupuncture, calming music, and laughter (especially good belly laughs) have all been shown to stimulate the production of nitric oxide—not to mention orgasms and having sex!

In turn, sufficient amounts of nitric oxide in the body seem to trigger positive emotions, including not only joy but also resilience, hardiness, and hope. Thus, pleasure boosts nitric oxide, and nitric oxide boosts pleasure. That's the upward spiral you should be aiming for!

The reason why nitric oxide acts as a bridge between your body and mind has to do with its unique ability to connect the usually unconnected parts of the brain that I talked about earlier in this chapter. If the "thinking" part of your brain is in a positive mind-set (because you're experiencing pleasure or are just plain thinking positive, uplifting thoughts), nitric oxide can then rapidly transmit positive signals to the "nonthinking" part of your brain. In response, the "nonthinking" part (which controls functions such as breathing and heart rate) sends out signals that decrease stress throughout your entire body. Nitric oxide also sends its life-affirming signals to the unconscious parts of your brain where instinct resides.

A good example of how all this works is the much-talked about placebo effect—the self-healing that occurs when you believe that a substance you're taking or a treatment you're given is an active medication or procedure, although it is actually totally inactive (such as a simple sugar pill or saline injection). The placebo effect isn't rare—researchers report that it occurs in anywhere from one-third of cases up to three-quarters of them.

Harvard Medical School mind-body medicine pioneer Herbert Benson, M.D., believes nitric oxide is the key to how and why the placebo effect works. The positive and hopeful emotions a patient feels when she's taking a medication she thinks might be beneficial trigger an increase in nitric oxide in her body, and the higher levels of nitric oxide in turn have a positive effect on her health—despite the fact that the medication contained no active ingredients.

Benson's research with nitric oxide goes further still. He suggests that higher levels of nitric oxide molecules in the brain can also trigger yearnings that lead us to having profound spiritual experiences.

So let's look at this all together: Creating sufficient levels of nitric oxide strengthens not just our physical health, but also our emotional and spiritual health.

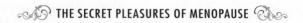

In other words, taking good care of your body and fully opening yourself to receiving pleasure (thus boosting nitric oxide) does all of the following:

- Helps the process of healing, boosts immunity, and helps prevent chronic degenerative diseases—keeping you physically strong and healthy as you age

- Improves not only your mood but also your outlook on life, renewing a sense of hope and strengthening your resolve to take charge of your health and your life

- Feeds your spirit, strengthening your sense of being a part of something much larger than yourself and possibly even leading to profound spiritual experiences

Ready to get started? I thought so!

CHAPTER FOUR

How to Achieve Maximal Levels of Life-Giving Nitric Oxide

Increasing your nitric oxide levels involves six important steps that engage your body, mind, and spirit. They are:

1. Associate yourself only with positive people everywhere you can.

2. Eat healthfully, exercise, and manage your weight.

3. Take pride in yourself!

4. Move forward—not backward!

5. Realize that you are what you believe.

6. Understand that sex and health go hand in hand.

You may have already mastered some of these steps, while others you may not have even considered yet. Know that wherever you are right now with these practices, it's important to keep reaching higher. This isn't something you can whip through in a weekend! Nor should you expect perfection from your efforts. Like so many other things in life, achieving these steps is a process. Expect to make progress and then slip back at times—it's only natural. Don't beat yourself up about it. The key is to move ahead over time and enjoy each step of the journey to its fullest!

1. Associate Yourself Only with Positive People Everywhere You Can

One of the most important and immediate ways to raise your levels of nitric oxide is to change the way you think. Thoughts are more than just words that flash through your mind. They are quite literally the power behind creating your reality (including your physical health). Thinking positive, optimistic thoughts is associated with higher levels of nitric oxide, which means a healthier you. The opposite is also true: Stress, chronic resentment, sadness, disappointment, fear, and anger decrease your levels of nitric oxide and can set you up for disease. Nothing good ever comes from undue stress.

One of the best ways to stay in this healthy, beneficial frame of mind is to surround yourself with like-minded people who will reinforce your choice to think positive thoughts. Remember the saying "Birds of a feather flock together"? It's true! Haven't you ever spent time with joyful, upbeat people who make you feel good just to be around them? It's almost like their mood is infectious. They make you feel lighter, happier, and more hopeful—even if your day started out crummy.

And the reverse is true as well. Spend time with someone who's negative, who always seems to be complaining about something, and who's always expecting the worst, and you'll start to feel as if a cloud is hanging over your head. You'll feel drained, exhausted, and pessimistic. Remember that like attracts like, so you can decide for yourself what sort of people and situations you want to surround yourself with.

This isn't to say that you should never grieve or get angry. Covering such normal, human emotions with a painted-on happy face isn't necessary and doesn't work. Nor am I suggesting that you become a sugar-sweet Pollyanna who lives in total denial—that's not good for your health either.

What I *am* suggesting is that you not get stuck in your negative feelings. (That's like sitting in your own dirty bath water for days!) Instead, feel *all* of your emotions—experience them fully and let them flow all the way through your body like a wave washing over you at the beach before it recedes back into the ocean.

We all face pain and disappointment. Stuff happens. But what crushes some people barely bothers others. Your ability to lead a healthy and happy life depends more on your perception of the events that unfold around you than on the actual events themselves. For example, seeing "problems" as challenges or opportunities for growth is an infinitely healthier perspective.

Simply put, your power to live a joyful, abundant, and vibrantly healthy life depends on how willing you are to focus your attention on thoughts, people, places, and experiences that are positive and uplifting. My motto is: "If it's not fun, don't do it!"

Let me give you a good example. If you say to yourself, *I am an incredibly sexy woman, and men [or women] find me desirable,* and you *believe* it (even just for a moment or two), here's what happens inside your body:

- Nitric oxide is released in the lining of your blood vessels, widening them to improve your circulation and deliver life-giving oxygen to every cell in your body faster.

- The circulation throughout your body is improved, including blood flow to your breasts and genitals, heightening your sexual experiences.

- Your levels of feel-good chemicals, such as serotonin and beta-endorphin, increase.

- The "nonthinking" part of your brain gets the signal that all is well, so it sends

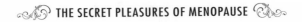

that message throughout your body, making you feel happier and more relaxed as well as optimizing your bodily functions, such as heart rhythm and tissue repair.

- Because you feel more attractive and desirable, you walk tall and talk in positive ways that make you more attractive and more desirable.

- You become a magnet for others who feel attractive and desirable, too. You also attract experiences validating that you are indeed attractive, sexy, and desirable to the universe. People notice you and smile, making *way* for you instead of bumping into you. They sense that you are vibrant and alive, and they want to be around you as much as possible.

Now if instead, you think on a regular basis, *I am old, unattractive, and over the hill; who would give me a second glance?* your experience will be quite different. Here's what happens then:

- Your levels of nitric oxide plummet, and stress hormones (such as cortisol and epinephrine) rise, increasing cellular inflammation. This eventually increases your chances of all degenerative diseases.

- The higher levels of cortisol adversely affect your blood sugar and insulin, leading to fatigue and weight gain. In fact, your "nonthinking" brain picks up your negative vibe and broadcasts signals to the rest of your body that encourage sluggishness and a lack of flow in all your systems. Things start to break down, including your immunity.

- Your eyes look dull and your steps are heavy. People tend to look right past you, not out of rudeness but simply because you don't engage their attention. You're broadcasting to the universe, *Don't mind dumpy old me,* so that's the experience you attract.

Which experience would you rather have? The fact is that when you *expect* good, you often *get* good. All the people you meet and the experiences you have can be seen as a reflection of your own inner beliefs. So if you don't like what life is dishing out, reprogram your state of mind. At least try it—it sure won't hurt, and you'll soon see how it works!

I've seen this many times in my own life. Five years ago, for example, I would have told you that there were no good men left—that all of them were married to women who are 20 years younger than they are. So whenever I did meet a man, his faults seemed magnified. What I didn't realize then was that all the flaws I noticed were really distorted reflections of the flaws I saw, or feared existed, in myself. Today, after shifting my viewpoint—starting with my perception about *myself* and my *own* desirability—I can sit next to any man and find at least two things about him to appreciate. And here's the best part: Men of all ages find more to appreciate about me, too! This never would have been possible if I hadn't first opened my heart to myself and taken the time to get into a more positive mind-set regularly. My new thoughts and attitude paved the way—with solid gold! And you can do it, too.

2. Eat Healthfully, Exercise, and Manage Your Weight

To boost your levels of nitric oxide, it's important to eat nutritious foods, maintain a healthy weight, get plenty of exercise, and take the right dietary supplements. If you've had trouble following this advice in the past, take heart. Sticking to a healthy lifestyle doesn't have to be torture, believe me! When your goal is to increase pleasure in your life instead of acting as a judgmental disciplinarian, the experience is completely different. You can indeed find healthy foods you enjoy eating and fun ways to get yourself moving. Once you begin to see some results, your self-esteem and your sexual desire will increase, and you'll be motivated to keep going. You'll live longer, too. Obesity is the number two preventable cause of death in the U.S. (right behind smoking). A study of more than 20,000 people published in 2008 in the U.K. reported that you can add an average of 14 years to your life by following a healthy lifestyle!

If you're very overweight, this can sometimes seem like an uphill battle. But be encouraged by the fact that losing even just 5 to 10 percent of your excess weight can decrease inflammation and improve your health. Remember, the goal here is to love yourself healthy, and you have to start somewhere! Avoid being too rigid; keep your sense of humor; and if you slip up, just get right back on track. Don't blame yourself or beat yourself up—that's counterproductive (and decreases nitric oxide).

Also be careful to set only healthy expectations. Don't fall prey to measuring yourself against an impossible (and unhealthy) cultural ideal. You're not trying to conform to society's standard. You're trying to be the healthiest *you* that you can be. So just do your best!

What to Eat

I want to be clear right from the start that I'm not suggesting you go on a diet. After all, the word *diet* has the word *die* in it. No wonder our bodies don't respond well to that term! I *am* suggesting that you adjust your lifestyle to make healthier choices that support your wellness by increasing your levels of nitric oxide. I want you to be able to *live* with and *love* what you choose to eat. You'll eventually find that the food you want the most is also the food that makes you feel the best.

What I've found that works the best and makes the most sense is a Mediterranean style of eating, traditionally followed in France, Italy, Greece, Spain, and Portugal—countries that have strikingly lower rates of cardiovascular disease compared to the U.S. And they're all countries that make pleasure a big part of the dining process! Basically, this involves eating fish, whole grains, fresh fruits and vegetables, legumes, nuts, and olive oil. It also means minimizing sugar, caffeine, junk food, and processed foods as much as possible.

Start with having five servings of fruits and veggies every day (one serving equals four ounces, or about one-half cup). Fresh rather than canned or frozen is always best—especially because processed foods generally contain sugar, salt, and other additives. Learn to read labels so that you can make the healthiest choices.

Moreover, not all vegetables are equal. Cut way back on starchy ones (such as potatoes and corn), in addition to white rice and anything made with white flour—including breads, muffins, bagels, biscuits, crackers, and pretzels. These foods are all heavy in high-glycemic carbs, which raise blood sugar and insulin levels too high, too fast. High blood sugar and subsequent high insulin not only decrease your nitric oxide, but these two factors also cause your body to store fat. You don't have to eliminate high-glycemic carbs completely, but eat them in moderation. And when you do eat them, choose the healthiest version. A baked potato is healthier than French fries, for example, and fresh corn on the cob doesn't have the added corn syrup that's in processed creamed corn. Oatmeal, quinoa, spelt, and millet are the best choices when you want grains and cereals. About one in four women is gluten intolerant (especially after age 50) and has far better digestion when avoiding wheat products.

Don't skimp on lean protein—it's an important part of any diet. Getting enough protein helps prevent carbohydrate cravings and increases glucagon, which jump-starts your body into burning fat. So make sure that you eat some with each meal and snack.

Many studies suggest that vegetable protein (for example, the protein found in beans) is healthier than animal protein, such as red meat. Yet in my experience, I've found that many people simply feel best with some red meat and other animal protein in their diet. I'm one of them. The healthiest source of animal protein is fish—especially mackerel, herring, salmon, trout, canned sardines in oil, and halibut, because these cold-water fish are high in heart-healthy omega-3 fats. Have fish at least two or three times a week. Organic chicken and turkey are other healthy sources of animal protein for those who don't want fish. Lean cuts of beef and pork come next. Game meats, such as venison and buffalo, are also naturally lean and healthy. Still other good sources of protein include organic eggs and dairy food. (Raw organic dairy products are the healthiest and most digestible because pasteurization destroys healthful enzymes.)

Cutting way down on sweets, junk food, and most processed food items is the most important thing you can do for several reasons. First of all, processed foods often contain unhealthy trans fats (often found in cookies, crackers, and other snack foods as well as in margarine and shortening), which increase cellular inflammation and decrease nitric oxide levels. Eating refined carbohydrates (such as candy, snack foods, and baked goods) is also damaging because it causes your blood sugar to spike and then crash. This can eventually lead to abnormal insulin levels, cellular inflammation, and (you guessed it) reduced nitric oxide. Healthier options for snacking include low-glycemic fruits (such as berries and pears) with low-fat cheese, low-glycemic nutritional bars, or a small handful of nuts (such as walnuts, almonds, or pecans—raw nuts are best).

Eating breakfast is another important key to keeping your blood-sugar levels stable, not just throughout the morning but for the whole day. If you aren't used to big breakfasts or don't have time to cook, don't worry! Just have a protein shake or meal-replacement bar—that's all it takes! Whatever you eat, make sure your breakfast includes some protein, low-glycemic-index carbohydrates (such as berries), and healthy fat.

Yes, there are healthy fats out there. (In fact, despite current conventional thinking, dietary fat—whether or not it's saturated—may not be the cause of obesity, heart disease, or any other disease of civilization. Refined carbs, especially sucrose and high-fructose corn syrup—which are just other types of sugar—are far more dangerous.) Fat is, in fact, required by every cell in your body. Your brain particularly relies on good fats for optimal health. The healthiest fats to eat are unsaturated—those that come mostly from plant sources or fish. Unsaturated fats include polyunsaturated fats (omega-3 and omega-6 fats, which come largely from fish, nuts, grains, and seeds) and monounsaturated fats (which also come from fish as well as olive oil, avocados, and nuts). Both monounsaturated and polyunsaturated fats are heart healthy and raise nitric oxide levels.

Although saturated fat (which generally comes from meat and dairy products) is not the culprit it's been made out to be, there are many good environmental reasons to limit saturated-fat consumption from animal sources. (Coconut oil, by the way, is a source of very healthy saturated fat.) Trans fats, however, which are found in margarine, shortening, and the processed products made from them, can be harmful to both heart health and nitric oxide levels.

Even if you can't keep all these recommendations in mind at once, make a commitment to start somewhere today. Then follow more and more of the plan as you feel comfortable doing so. I guarantee you, once you've eaten this way for even just a few days (especially if your diet right now includes a lot of refined foods), you'll be amazed by how much better you'll feel and by how much more energy you'll have once you've adopted this new plan! I know that this has made a huge difference for me!

I also want to suggest that you drink lots of water every day. A good guideline is to drink half your body weight in ounces daily. (If you weigh 140 pounds, for example, drink 70 ounces of water a day, which is a little more than half a gallon or a bit more than a two-liter bottle.) Water is important for keeping your entire body working smoothly (including burning fat). When you feel thirsty, your body is already dehydrated! So don't wait until you're thirsty to drink—keep a water bottle with you and take sips all day long. Also remember that thirst is sometimes mistaken for hunger. Next time you get a hunger pang, take a sip of water before reaching for that snack!

By the way, coffee and other caffeinated drinks (such as colas) aren't a good substitute for water because caffeine increases blood sugar and cellular inflammation. You should also limit your alcohol intake. Alcohol in moderation won't harm you, but remember that nutritionally speaking, it's nothing but empty calories and sugar that goes straight to your brain. (Hence the saying, "Candy is dandy, but liquor is quicker.")

Finally, pay attention to *when* you eat. Because your metabolic rate naturally peaks at noon (and slows down later in the day), it's best to avoid eating late at night. Night eating not only packs on the pounds faster, but it can also make your blood sugar unstable. Sometimes a small snack around 4 P.M. (if you feel the need) can keep you from overeating at dinner as well as later at night. Eating breakfast also helps prevent nighttime hunger!

One final thought on diet: Your thoughts and emotions directly and powerfully affect how your food gets digested. For example, when you're in love, you often feel satisfied with much less food and can also lose weight easily. The take-home message is to enjoy your food thoroughly—and cultivate the pleasurable art of dining well!

Get Moving!

To a lot of women, exercise is a dirty word. So if you don't enjoy going to the gym, don't go. If you hate sit-ups, never do another one again. But I *do* want you to move your body in some form that you enjoy on a regular basis. Find something that's fun, whether it's jogging, tennis, Pilates, yoga, biking, hula hooping, spinning, gardening, or just dancing yourself silly around the house. Exercise can be empowering—it doesn't have to be intimidating. What matters most is that you find something that you love enough to do regularly. You'll soon get hooked—especially when you see how good (and sexy) it makes you feel and how great your body looks as a result.

Here's why it's so important: As you age, if you don't get enough exercise, your muscle mass is often replaced by fat. Once you start an exercise program, no matter what your age, you can reverse that trend.

Even more important, women who exercise regularly have an average of 20 more years of productive living than those who don't. That's because regular exercise helps regulate weight and decreases insulin resistance, boosting nitric oxide. It also keeps all your joints mobile and lubricated.

Actually, all you really need is just 20 to 30 minutes of aerobic exercise (like brisk walking—enough to get you huffing and puffing) at least five days a week. More is even better! Also do some form of strength training (with weights, resistance bands, or Pilates equipment) three times a week. Strength training is vital because it's the only type of exercise that can slow the muscle and bone losses many women start to experience in midlife. You don't have to go to the gym for this—you can use handheld weights (or resistance bands) at home. If you're new to weights, however, it's a good idea to hire a trainer at least in the beginning so that you can get advice on what routine to follow and how to do it safely.

Respect your limits and rest (or stop) when you need to. If you feel depleted afterward (not just tired but *worn out*), you've gone too far and have done too much. It's best to start out slowly and build on your routine. One way to stay motivated (and interested) is to set regular and reasonable goals, like walking around the block or to a particular destination in less and less time, or adding five to ten minutes to your routine each week or so. Pedometers are especially motivating. Try working up to 10,000 steps per day.

Catch Enough Z's

Getting sufficient sleep is also important for keeping nitric oxide levels high. Many women (including me!) require eight to ten hours of sleep for optimal functioning, but you may need slightly more or slightly less. The test is simple: If you're groggy and tired throughout the day, you need more sleep! Recent studies indicate that sleep deprivation contributes greatly to high blood pressure and even weight gain.

If you can, get to bed by 10 P.M. Falling asleep before midnight is healthier for your body than sleep that begins later in the night—even if you sleep in later the next morning. And believe it or not, getting the right amount of sleep can also help you lose weight!

Kick the Habit

If you smoke, quit. End of story. Smoking is the number one cause of preventable death in America, and it substantially lowers your nitric oxide levels. Find some support (either with a stop-smoking program, hypnosis, or by using a nicotine patch), but stop for good. Believe me, it's well worth it, and after a while, you'll wonder what took you so long!

Supplements

We can't always get the nutrients we need from food, so to be sure you're getting what you need, take supplements. Pick a high-quality supplement from a reputable manufacturer. Look for the NSF (The Public Health and Safety Company™) or the USP (United States Pharmacopeia) logo on the label. Check the dosage carefully, because you can't get optimal supplementation from merely one pill per day. You'll usually have to take at least four daily, and possibly more. Shoot for a supplement with the following daily levels per dose:

- Beta-carotene: 2,500–15,000 IU
- Thiamin (B_1): 20–40 mg

- Riboflavin (B$_2$): 20–40 mg
- Niacin (B$_3$): 20–40 mg
- Pantothenic Acid (B$_5$): 20–100 mg
- Pyridoxine (B$_6$): 20–35 mg
- Vitamin B$_{12}$: 100–600 mcg
- Folic Acid: 400–1,000 mcg
- Vitamin C: 1,000–2,000 mg
- Vitamin D$_3$: 600–2,000 IU
- Vitamin E: 200–400 IU
- Calcium: 650–1,200 mg
- Selenium: 200 mcg
- Magnesium: 400–1,000 mg
- Zinc: 20–40 mg
- Chromium: 100–300 mcg
- Biotin: 30–300 mcg
- Boron: 3–5 mg
- CoQ10: 10–200 mg
- Fish Oil/Omega-3: 200–1,500 mg of DHA and 400–1,850 mg of EPA
- Lutein: 500–1,000 mcg
- Lycopene: 500–1,000 mcg

Optional:

- Glutathione: 2–10 mg
- Alpha Lipoic Acid: 10–100 mg
- Inositol: 10–500 mg

- Choline: 10–100 mg
- Manganese: 1–15 mg
- Copper: 1–2 mg
- Molybdenum: 10–25 mcg
- Vanadium: 20–40 mcg

Remember, your body doesn't naturally manufacture most of the vitamins and minerals that you require. *Note:* The RDA (recommended daily allowance) that was set up by the USDA was designed as a guideline to prevent gross deficiency diseases; optimal nutrition requires higher nutrient levels.

3. Take Pride in Yourself!

As I've already mentioned, the number one predictor of a great sex life after menopause is a new partner. Now don't get excited . . . read on! This is proof positive that there's nothing about menopause, per se, that results in an "equipment failure." And this doesn't mean that you need to get a divorce or leave your current partner in order to have red-hot sex! Here's the great news: You can *become* that new partner yourself! And in the process, you can wake up all the desire and pleasure that your body is capable of experiencing.

Remember that perimenopause is a turning point in your life, a huge biologically supported opportunity to reinvent yourself and experience more joy and pleasure than you've ever dreamed possible. At this time when you're reevaluating your life and deciding what works and what doesn't, you get a chance to start with a clean slate. The best way to do so is to have fun with the process. Make yourself over anyway you want. Let your imagination (and your desire) go wild!

If you've always wanted to try a different hair color, for example, now is your time to go for it. Maybe try a different hairstyle (or three—why stop with just one?). Or perhaps you want to change the way you dress, trying colors and styles that you've never worn before. Experiment with what clothes and accessories feel and look good. How about outrageously entertaining earrings? Here's a particularly fun idea: Buy all new underwear, and don't let any of it be "sensible"! Nobody has to know but you—and hopefully your partner! The main thing to remember is that the person you must turn on first is *you*. This is the key not only to great sex, but also to vibrant health.

If you're at all intimidated by these ideas (most of us are at the beginning), start small—just start somewhere.

When I first wore an oversized velour leopard-print shirt after my divorce, my youngest daughter thought I was out of my mind. But I loved it!

(*Note:* When you're reinventing yourself, especially your sensual self, it's quite common for your children to be embarrassed by your new look or behavior. Don't let this stop you. The biggest gift you can give to your kids is your own personal fulfillment and happiness. You are a role model to them for what their future selves will look like. Give them a role model who is fully alive, sensual, and empowered. Trust me, as time goes on, they'll love you for it.)

Back at the beginning of my own midlife reinvention, that leopard-print shirt was about as far as I was willing to go. But after about four or five years, I totally transformed my wardrobe. Remember, your new look and style is all about entertaining yourself—whether or not anyone else sees it! (It's also helpful to have a trusted friend gently push you in a new, more youthful direction in this regard.)

"Mirror, Mirror"

Here's something else I want you to do that can make a powerful difference. I call it the *mirror exercise.* Stand in front of a mirror twice a day for 30 days, and look deeply into your eyes. As you do so, say out loud: "I accept myself unconditionally right now." (If you'd like to get on the fast track right away, add, "I love you. You're fabulous!") Spend time admiring yourself in the mirror and looking at yourself with truly loving eyes, the way you'd lovingly gaze at a puppy or a small child. This isn't a time to inspect for flaws, sagging skin, or new wrinkles. It's a time to appreciate how great your skin looks, your beautiful eye color, the warmness of your smile, and so on. Perhaps even more important, this is a time to look at what you might otherwise find fault with and instead see it in a new light. At first, this mirror exercise will seem silly and maybe even stupid. It will also alert your inner critic who will pop into your head with put-downs. Expect this—and don't let it stop you. The mirror exercise is very powerful for healing and transformation.

When you look at your abdomen, for example, instead of thinking it's saggy or fat, think to yourself, *This belly held and nourished each of my children for many months. What joy that belly has brought me—and the rest of the world! I love my belly!* And if you haven't given birth, love your curves just because they're yours! When you see your legs, think to yourself, *I'm so lucky to have good strong legs that can walk, dance, stretch, support, and carry me through anything. These are great legs!*

What you're doing is actually seeing yourself with *new* eyes. And the more you enjoy your body and yourself, the more sexy and erotic you'll feel. As Sophia Loren once said, "Nothing makes a woman more beautiful than the belief that she is beautiful." After all, feeling sexy starts as an *inside* job.

Even if the mirror exercise seems awkward at first, stick with it. It will get easier in time, especially when you see how positive the results of this are. Granted, society doesn't make it easy for women to love their bodies. Most of us compare ourselves to the stick-thin models and celebrities whose carefully crafted and air-brushed images are plastered all over the media every day. But chances are, your body's normal, healthy size is larger than the bodies you view on television and in magazines. After all, most fashion models are thinner than 98 percent of American women. That's gotta tell you something! So instead of scrutinizing your figure with a critical eye, learn to look at it with a loving eye and embrace it.

Here's another important point: Don't motivate yourself by thinking that you're doing this exercise to feel sexy for your partner. Although your partner will undoubtedly benefit from you loving and appreciating your body and feeling sexier, you're doing this for *yourself*. You're learning a new way to see and speak to yourself. You're learning a new way to *love* yourself. And with every genuinely loving, appreciative thought, you're bathing your body in more and more nitric oxide. And by the way, most men are far more accepting of women's bodies than we women ourselves.

Pampering Makes Perfect

Pamper yourself during this transition time, too—especially if you're not used to doing so. Take more bubble baths. Get manicures and pedicures and admire how lovely your hands and feet look afterward, appreciating how good it feels to be pampered a little. Don't wait for a special occasion either! One friend of mine made a ritual out of lovingly massaging her feet every night with incredibly fragrant peppermint foot cream. She said at first it felt funny and terribly self-indulgent to caress her feet like that, but she very quickly came to love the ritual! (And her feet did, too!)

Go to a department store cosmetics counter and ask for a makeover. Try a different scent—something you wouldn't ordinarily try. While we're talking pampering, why not treat yourself to a massage? Think of it as anointing yourself as you go through this initiation into a new stage in your life, because that's exactly what midlife is!

Instead of lamenting the loss of your youth, this initiation is about celebrating the fact that you're nearing or are over 50 (or 60, 70, 80, or 90) and are still actively engaged in life, with a healthy, beautiful, and sexy body that deserves some special treatment. When you can give yourself this kind of loving attention and know from the deepest part of you that you fully deserve it, you'll be open to receiving loving attention from others—including your husband or partner. Remember, receiving is a skill that has to be developed. The more you learn how to receive, the more pleasure you'll be able to attract and experience. You can start by saying thank you to all compliments!

Cue Your Creativity!

Another vital part of making yourself over and opening to your true essence involves surrounding yourself with beauty and deliberately using your creativity.

Rearrange things in your home, or maybe get new furniture or repaint. Your home is a direct extension of your innermost self. That's why women dream about houses all the time. At midlife, as they redo themselves at the deepest levels, many women also have an insatiable urge to redo their homes as well!

I know a woman, for example, who never had anything but neutral colored walls in her house until she got divorced at midlife. After her husband moved out, she painted her bedroom a soothing, uplifting yellow and made drapes that matched perfectly. She also bought a new bedspread with beautifully coordinating pillow covers. Every time she walked into that room, she thought to herself, *Wow!* And every time she thought (and felt) that *wow,* it was an affirmation that she not only felt good in that room, but that she felt good in her new life.

Buy yourself armfuls of fresh flowers and put them in several rooms in your home where you can see them often. Play music you love more often (and maybe try some new music to see what else you might enjoy). If someone made a movie of your life from this day forward, what music would you want to be on the soundtrack? Play that!

Buy some new art and display it prominently. Better yet, *create* some new art for your home (or even to give to others). This is a time in life when your creative juices are ready and willing to flow like never before, even if you haven't previously thought of yourself as very creative. Try writing in a journal. Studies have shown that writing down your feelings is associated with healing of all kinds. Who knows, you may also get a great idea for an article or even a book! Painting, sculpting, or learning to play an instrument are also good choices. Many women also return to activities they loved in the past—such as horseback riding, roller skating, or ice skating. You might take a cooking class and invite friends over to sample the results. Or take photos of more than just family gatherings. If you like sending detailed e-mails to friends, start your own blog. Don't limit your singing to the shower anymore! Hint: What did you love to do when you were 11? This holds a clue to what would nourish you now.

If you already enjoy creative projects, experiment with giving them a bit of a twist. If you like writing, try poetry. If you are good at needlework, try sewing. A colleague of mine had a mother who was an incredibly talented seamstress. When she hit midlife, she stopped making clothing and started making teddy bears (each with an outrageously funny name), dressing them in hilarious outfits complete with carefully chosen accessories. Her creativity was totally reborn!

While you're being creative, why not take a belly-dancing class? Or try pole dancing or erotic dancing. That's right—move your body in totally new ways. Why not? You might be pleasantly surprised! After all, there's no better way to learn to love your body *and* feel sexy at the same time. The idea behind all of these suggestions is to stretch your perceptions of who you are and what you can do because you're giving birth to an entirely new self. These classes are ladies only, so you get a great deal of support from other women. And when you're birthing a new self, this support is crucial—as is the support of like-minded friends.

Don't be upset if you're not really good at something you try for the first time or if you decide you're really not the red-lace underwear type. The point is to have fun finding your best self. Dolly Parton put it this way: "Find out who you are, and do it on purpose." Keep pushing your boundaries and enjoying the process. You'll be absolutely amazed by the new you waiting to be discovered!

4. Move Forward—Not Backward!

Rebirthing yourself and embracing a new way of life entails letting go of the past as well. It's like cleaning out your closets—when you throw out or give away the stuff you no longer want (or which no longer expresses who you're becoming), you have plenty of room to accumulate new things that you need and will appreciate more. So as you enter this new phase of life, see it as the perfect opportunity to let go of relationships, behaviors, and beliefs (including thoughts and beliefs about unhealed emotional wounds) that hold you back and don't support the new you who is now being born. To create vibrant health, you must move forward, not backward!

Letting the Past Pass

Letting go of the past is vital because staying hung up on prior hurts and disappointments means that you're not living fully in the present. And if you're not in the present, you can't create a healthy and happy future! You can't do anything to change the past, so rehashing in your mind what was said or done won't get you anywhere. In fact, carrying resentment—as with most negative emotions—puts stress on your physical body, increasing cellular inflammation, weakening the immune system over time, and decreasing nitric oxide levels.

Although you can't change the past, you probably *can* do something (no matter how small) right now to make your life work better. After all, it's only in the present that you can become empowered and take action. So thinking about what you *can* do or change, rather than what you *can't* do, gets you unstuck and keeps you moving forward. If you're upset about a perceived wrong someone has perpetrated upon you, ask yourself if you'd rather be right or . . . healthy and happy. And then make healthy and happy happen! Remember, it isn't so much what life dishes out to you that determines how content you are; it has more to do with how you react to and deal with the events and circumstances that come your way.

You'll probably have lots of opportunities to practice this "letting go of the past" at midlife because so many unhealed emotions tend to surface at this stage. Everything seems to be in your face all the time. But as uncomfortable as that may seem, look at it this way: This is a fabulous chance to heal what needs healing and move on, once and for all. It's all part of the labor pains of birthing the new you.

When you were a kid, did you ever play with magic slates—those pads with a black waxy surface covered by a gray plastic sheet? You could write on the sheet using a pointed stylus, and then as soon as you lifted up the plastic sheet, what you'd written disappeared. You were left with a clean slate—literally. That's what you're aiming for here—erasing the dark marks of the past, leaving a fresh, clean slate full of potential.

Your Prescription for Forgiveness

Practicing forgiveness regularly is a great way to keep that slate clean! This is possible even when the person you're angry with is dead or otherwise not reachable. Here's what you have to know: Forgiveness is all about you, not the other person. Forgiving someone simply means that you are no longer willing to allow what happened in the past to adversely affect you now. Sometimes it's possible to work out your differences with the person you have a grievance with and begin again. But this isn't always possible or even advisable. Instead, you must have the courage to forgive and let go.

This is a process, not an event—especially if the wound is something like childhood abuse by a parent. When it comes to lesser grievances, such as a misunderstanding with a boss or friend, I want you to notice something: If you look back five years ago, I'll bet you'll discover that there are many relationships that have simply gone by the wayside. As you grow and change, you quite naturally "outgrow" some of the people in your life—especially those who have hurt you in some way. This is natural and good.

Destructive relationships often spur your most important growth. That's the basis of the saying "Strong in the broken places." But you can't get strong—and experience vibrant health and pleasure— if you're still hanging on to the past, waiting for someone else to validate or take away your pain. As an adult, you have to be responsible to yourself.

A really good way to forgive someone is to set up two chairs facing each other. Imagine yourself sitting opposite the person you have a grievance with and having a heart-to-heart conversation, getting everything off your chest. This alone moves energy and is healing. Another powerful method is to write a letter to the angel of the individual you're resenting, pouring out everything in your heart—how the person has hurt you, how angry you are, and so forth—and then stating what you'd like to see happen. Then burn the letter. I've seen this work miracles!

A woman I know had an alcoholic father who was physically and emotionally abusive to her and her mother. She had an incredible amount of anger built up toward him because of the abuse, and it seemed perfectly justified to her because of the horrible things he'd done. Yet she couldn't seem to release that rage—even though her father had been dead for 20 years, her mother was remarried to a loving husband, and she herself was happily married with three children.

Finally one night, directed by a meditation she was doing with friends, she pictured her father not as the raging, drunken adult she had always known him to be, but as a little boy. During the meditation, she saw in this little boy's face the pain and agony that he felt growing up with *his* parents, and she could envision the origin of his wanting to escape with alcohol before it had actually happened. She imagined herself holding this wounded boy, who now seemed more like a victim than a perpetrator. She comforted him and rocked him, soothing him and making him feel loved and safe.

Nurturing and protecting this frightened little boy in her imagination seemed to come as naturally to her in the meditation as did mothering her own children in real life. When the meditation was over, she realized that while she still felt that the abuse her father dished out to her and her mother was very wrong, she no longer felt as angry toward him. She had taken a huge step in forgiving him. She felt lighter, more free—and better able to focus on her present life rather than dwell in the past.

An important key to forgiveness is not allowing yourself to feel like a victim any longer. If you're used to wearing your wounds on your sleeve, it's time to take off the victim armband and toss it away! Eleanor Roosevelt once said, "No one can make you feel inferior without your consent." Similarly, no one can make you feel victimized if you don't allow it. Thank heaven for that!

"I Forgive You, *but . . .*"

Sometimes you can believe that you've forgiven someone else, but you're really still caught in the past, holding on to your resentment. That happens when you forgive in your head (which means you've basically talked yourself into it) but your heart isn't fully onboard with that decision. A good test of this is the following: If you find yourself saying that you've forgiven this person for saying this or for doing that, *but* . . . then you haven't really forgiven. Full forgiveness doesn't come with a *but*. If you forgive, you forgive. End of story. No buts.

To truly forgive (and to get the full benefit of the higher levels of nitric oxide that come when you let go of your negativity), you must forgive not only in your head, but also from your heart. This is a very important distinction because the electromagnetic field of your heart (which is the center of your emotions) is hundreds of times more powerful than the electromagnetic field of your brain (the center of your thoughts). It means that no matter what you *think*, what you *feel* always wins—always!

But how do you get there? Again it comes down to deciding if you'd rather be right or be healthy and happy. You must make up your mind. As the woman struggling with forgiving her alcoholic father discovered, right and wrong aren't always so cut and dried. Human beings are complex creatures, and the situations we find ourselves in are rarely all black or all white.

For as long as possible, look at the situation from your compassionate heart, resisting the urge to allow your judgmental thoughts to take over. And then instead of focusing on what is wrong in any given memory or situation, you'll be naturally more inclined to give your attention to what right and loving action you can take. The more you focus on that, the more you're able to stay in the present and make progress. And the more you work on forgiveness, the easier it will become. Trust me!

Forgiving Yourself

I've been talking about forgiving other people, but the fact is that quite often, the person you most need to pardon is yourself. Women are so good at beating themselves up for falling short of some ridiculously idealistic benchmark—not being thin enough, sexy enough, smart enough, clever enough, loving enough, strong enough. Chances are, you're harder on yourself than on anyone else in your life! But berating yourself doesn't ever do any good—all it does is make you feel worse about yourself. It won't ever help you make any positive change. And it certainly isn't good for your nitric oxide levels!

Whenever you find yourself being overly self-critical or abusive, try this exercise. Imagine your higher self, your guardian angel, or some other Divine figure standing in front of you. See this light-filled being as radiating total love and compassion.

See her reaching out and putting her hand on the top of your head as she calls you by name and says:

"I now forgive you for all the times that you ate too much ice cream, lost your temper, didn't clean your house, let the laundry pile up, misplaced something important, arrived too late, or didn't keep your promises to yourself or someone else. I forgive you for being human, for not being perfect, and for not being able to make everyone around you happy all the time. I forgive you for ever doubting your worth or feeling afraid."

Then allow that feeling of forgiveness to seep through your skin, into your body, and all the way into your heart. Feel it radiating throughout your entire body. Feel yourself being engulfed in the loving light of forgiveness. And as you do so, know that you are also bathing your heart and your body in the energy of perfect health.

Feel free to practice this exercise or any forgiveness exercise anytime you need to. Remember that forgiveness is a process, so as bad feelings surface, you'll need to work on releasing them one by one. Here's a self-forgiveness ritual that I recommend you do for 40 days. Light a candle and say a prayer of your choice. Then say out loud: "I now forgive myself for everything that I didn't know or do in the past. I release myself to my highest joy and purpose in life."

Try not to judge the process, just stick with it. Think of this as cleaning your emotional house. Now that you've gotten rid of all the junk that's been piling up in there, feel the energy of the sunlight pouring into the freshly washed windows and filling the rooms. Feels good, doesn't it? And now *you* can feel good, from the inside out!

5. Realize That You Are What You Believe

Ignoring harmful menopausal myths will help you experience maximum pleasure (sexual and otherwise) at midlife and beyond. The first idea you need to cast aside is the cultural myth that sex drive inevitably decreases after menopause. This is simply not true. The latest research shows that women in their 60s and 70s have the best sex of their lives. And so can you!

For example, a much-talked-about survey of 3,000 men and women ranging in age from 57 to 85 was published in *The New England Journal of Medicine* in 2007. Not only were most of those surveyed still sexually active, but the average frequency of sex was two to three times a month—the same frequency that younger adults report. Even among the oldest group surveyed (75- to 85-year-olds), more than a quarter were still having sex!

The survey also showed that those in poor health reported the least action between the sheets, while those who said they were healthy reported the most. The bottom line, the researchers note, is that having sex has *less* to do with how old you are and *more* to do with how healthy you are. And since you're now focusing on raising your nitric oxide levels and improving your health, that's very good news indeed for you!

Here's more good news: Not only are midlife adults having sex more often, but they're also enjoying it more than ever before. Proof comes in a report from an ongoing study on midlife change that was given at the annual meeting of the Gerontological Society of America in 2007. The report revealed that U.S. women aged 55 and older enjoy sex more and put more thought and effort into their sex lives than women the same age a decade ago. Those in their mid-60s to mid-70s reported the biggest increase!

The researchers conducting the study explain the difference in this way: Women who've reached midlife and beyond feel younger, are more open about their sexual needs, and are more interested in health than women at the same age a decade ago. Not only that, but today's midlife women see a healthy sex life as being part of a healthy lifestyle.

But there's even more to it than that. The second half of life offers an unparalleled opportunity to create the best sex of your life because truly great sex (for both men and women) happens in the context of genuine intimacy. (Remember, *intimacy* stands for INTO ME SEE.) Intimate relationships are characterized by commitment, trust, and vulnerability. In the second half of life, many men get in touch with their nurturing side in a whole new way—and this makes greater intimacy possible, perhaps for the first time. That's why so many committed couples say that their best years together have occurred after the age of 50—despite the fact that their bodies are no longer young! As relationship expert Harville Hendrix, Ph.D., explains, both men and women can become healers for each other. What a wonderful thing to look forward to!

A New Perspective on Midlife

The simple truth is that there's *nothing* about perimenopause or menopause that inevitably decreases either your sex drive or how often you can have an orgasm. Those problems that do crop up can usually be easily addressed. For example, if you experience vaginal dryness that makes intercourse or other sexual activities uncomfortable, you can use a little dab of estrogen cream as prescribed by your healthcare practitioner or any of several lubricants widely available in pharmacies. Problem solved!

If you find your libido lagging, you might simply need to take some time to become acquainted with your newly emerging self and to give yourself the opportunity to reassess your goals and current relationships. This libido lag is quite common, and it's also quite temporary! It's merely your body's way of making sure that you give yourself the time and space you need to do some inner work. (This is especially true if you discover that a lot of previously suppressed emotional issues are now emerging.) You'll find yourself back "in the mood" again before too long.

Even if you've had a hysterectomy or you've had your ovaries removed, you're not out of the game by a long shot. A little prescription hormonal support could work wonders for you, but that isn't always necessary—you might not need supplemental hormones at all to feel sexual. One of my 50-something friends is a good example. Ten years ago, she was treated for breast cancer with a lumpectomy, chemotherapy, radiation, and the removal of her uterus and ovaries. She's now enjoying more pleasure in her life than ever before—and that includes sexual pleasure. The only hormonal support she needs is some vaginal estrogen in the form of a prescription silicone ring (sold as Estring) that's placed in the vagina. (Always discuss estrogen use after breast cancer with your personal physician, because generally it's not recommended, even though I personally believe that in many instances, it's perfectly safe.)

"It was the decision to allow myself to feel pleasure that changed everything," she told me. "That decision is what jump-started my libido—and also increased my vaginal lubrication significantly." (Nitric oxide strikes again!) As my friend's story illustrates, having a good relationship with your partner (and yourself) as well as having a strong life force is often enough to change your hormone levels. So kicking up your nitric oxide levels could be all that you need to heat up your sex life!

After all, great sex always begins in the mind. The brain is the biggest and most important sex organ in the body—and that's true whether you're 28 or 88! What it means for you is this: If you think of yourself as a sexual being, your body will indeed comply with this image and respond accordingly. You will feel sexual, act sexual, and think sexual. So be it! I've seen it over and over again—it's true. The biggest hurdle to having a hot sex life can be as simple as accepting that it is indeed possible to have fabulous sex after menopause *and* believing that you deserve it!

A word about hormone therapy (which used to be called hormone replacement therapy, or HRT): Some women do feel better on hormone therapy. If you've tried everything and still find your libido flagging, I recommend getting your hormone levels checked and then starting on a low dose of bioidentical estradiol, progesterone, and/or testosterone. Hormone therapy is an art as well as a science, and it can take a while to ascertain the right dosage for you.

In general, I prefer a transdermal approach where you apply hormone preparations to your skin. This produces a more natural effect than taking hormone pills does. Avoid synthetic hormones that aren't native to the human female body, which include Premarin, Provera, and Prempro. Many other preparations are widely available. (For further information, please read the hormone section of my book *The Wisdom of Menopause* or log on to **www.drnorthrup.com**.)

The hundreds of thousands of women who are marching into their midlife years during this era are passionately redefining cultural expectations—including the expectations about midlife sexuality. Think of it this way: You're quite likely to live 30 to 40 years or more after menopause, so this truly is the "springtime" of the second half of your life.

I'm a good example. I led a full and wonderful life before I hit menopause. But since my transition to midlife has been complete, my life has far exceeded all my expectations in every way! My capacity for joy has expanded exponentially. Physically, I've not only lost weight, but I've also become more flexible and healthier than ever. And I've *never* felt sexier! If it can happen for me, it can happen for you, too.

Remember that the only person who can stand in the way of you seeing yourself as an incredibly sexy woman is *you!*

Being Your Own Better Half

Another perspective that needs updating is the idea that you need a man (or a mate) to be happy. That's nonsense! Not having a partner doesn't mean that you're any less sexy, any less desirable, or any less able to create exquisite joy and pleasure in your life (and in the lives of others). While having a partner can be an extremely fulfilling experience, and one you may very well want, it isn't the case that you *need* a partner in order to be a whole woman.

When you look to another to make yourself whole, you'll inevitably be disappointed. No one can stoke your life force but *you*. You make it happen. Only you can know your own truth, and only you can dialogue with your very soul.

I suggest you begin this part of your journey by defining yourself as a sex *subject* rather than a sex *object*—meaning that you see yourself not primarily as a vehicle for providing pleasure to others, but as a woman who is fully able to bring herself pleasure and joy, all on her own. This paradigm shift is not only revolutionary, it's downright evolutionary! To accomplish it, you must be willing to take control of your own life, becoming the commander of your own destiny. Forget about being a damsel still waiting around for Prince Charming to arrive and make your dreams come true. *You* must make your own happiness and pleasure a priority.

At first, that might sound a bit crazy and even selfish. It certainly bucks convention, doesn't it? But when you realize beyond a shadow of a doubt that you're not only *able* to create your own pleasure, but that you're also *responsible* for it, you'll stop being disappointed in (and angry with) other people who either can't or won't do it for you. This doesn't mean that no one else can bring you joy and pleasure. They certainly can! But when you take responsibility for giving yourself what you want and need (as well as making requests of others, when appropriate), you'll feel more in control of your life and less like a victim at the mercy of the whims of others. Taking this step is deliciously empowering!

Here's why: When you begin bringing joy into your own life instead of expecting someone else to deliver it (or to give you permission to have it), you'll start every day and every interaction from a healthier and more balanced, positive, loving, and giving place. Because you won't have your hand out, you'll be able to give others a hand up. You'll be better able than ever before to give from your heart, without expectation of return. And when you can do that, the joy you experience as a result is unlimited. It's a paradox: Those who give the most (from a full heart) end up receiving the most. And now that you're at midlife, you have an opportunity to understand this and see the effects it has on your body and mind in a whole new way.

Opening to the Spiritual

When you begin consciously bringing more pleasure into your life, you not only experience profound joy, but you also open the door to experiencing what can only be described as spiritual ecstasy. This is possible because you're certainly more than your physical body: You are a physical *and* a spiritual being. And just as your mind and body are intimately connected, you're also intimately connected with Source Energy. No matter what you call it—your Higher Self, Spirit, God, Goddess—Source Energy is the greater whole that we're all a part of.

When you drop the garbage you're holding (all those self-limiting thoughts and outmoded ideas) and allow yourself to accept and then really feel the unlimited joy and passion that's waiting for you, you'll feel your connection with Source Energy more strongly than ever. This powerful connection doesn't merely make you feel good, it feeds your very soul. It's like a spiritual orgasm! Goddess energy, the feminine face of Source Energy, never ages. *Ever.* Isn't that wonderful?

It shouldn't be surprising then that when you feel more Source Energy flowing within you, when that uplifting ecstatic energy starts spiking, the experience is often quite erotic. After all, pleasure breeds more pleasure. So ladies, fasten your seatbelts!

6. Understand That Sex and Health Go Hand in Hand

Sexual ecstasy isn't a luxury; rather, it's vitally important to your vibrant health for a number of reasons. In fact, the two go hand in hand. To understand why, you must first recognize that sex doesn't just happen below your waist—sexual ecstasy is a full-body experience. And even more than that, it's a mind-body event. So when you add more on one side of the equation, it makes sense that the other side would end up with more, too.

For example, there's a real connection between what I call your "low heart" (your uterus, pelvis, genitals, and that whole area of your body) and what I call your "high heart" (your physical heart muscle as well as the seat of all your emotions). Having sex that involves your body and emotions results in maximum pleasure (which may well mean orgasm, but could also be any intensely enjoyable physical sensation). But that isn't the end of the story. Connecting your low and high hearts by experiencing sexual ecstasy on a regular basis leads to optimum pleasure on an even *grander* level—a more physically, emotionally, and spiritually healthy you!

The late Earle Marsh, M.D., of the Institute for Advanced Study of Human Sexuality in San Francisco (and the famous author of the "Physician, Heal Thyself" story in what members of Alcoholics Anonymous call *The Big Book*) put it this way:

> If people would get more sensually involved with those they care for, they would have less illness, would sleep better and there would be fewer of them in hospitals or in an early grave! Hugging, touching, kissing, anything like that would do! We have found that sex is one of the most efficient treatments in relieving tension, which is the root cause of so many ailments. Once the tension is gone, then the intimacy of sex continues to cure and remove all the symptoms. Sex, even just intimate bodily contact, works to bring relief to the whole body!

I've seen this borne out again and again in my own life as well as in the lives of others. The concept came up again recently when I spoke at a session of Mama Gena's School of Womanly Arts in New York City. Regena Thomashauer (aka Mama Gena) is all about teaching women to experience more joy and pleasure by saying yes to themselves and their lives. Before I started my talk, I asked if any of the women gathered there had experienced a healing or an improvement in a health condition while taking Mama Gena's class. More than a dozen hands shot up.

Each of the women then shared with the group how deliberately cultivating more pleasure in their lives had helped them achieve more vibrant health, reversing or at least greatly improving debilitating conditions such as lupus and migraine headaches that many people struggle with for decades. Hearing their stories was incredibly inspiring. My initial hunch was correct: The deliberate cultivation of more pleasure in life actually helps heal the body.

How Sex Keeps You Healthy

Let me give you some specific examples of how sex creates health. First of all, as I mentioned in Chapter 3, sexual pleasure is associated with the release of nitric oxide from the lining of your blood vessels. The release of nitric oxide helps blood flow more easily to all your vital organs, reducing high blood pressure and decreasing cellular inflammation.

Decreasing cellular inflammation is significant because this inflammation leads to various chronic degenerative diseases, including killers such as heart disease, strokes, cancer, and diabetes, as well as asthma, arthritis, Alzheimer's disease, autoimmune disease, digestive disorders, hormonal imbalances, osteoporosis, and Parkinson's.

There's even scientific evidence for the link between the frequency of sex and longevity. Researchers from Queen's University in Belfast studied 918 men living in South Wales and ranging in age from 45 to 59 for ten years to see if there was any relationship between frequency of sex and heart disease. In a 1997 edition of the revered *British Medical Journal,* researchers asserted that the more sex the men in the study had, the longer they lived. Those who reported having sex at least three times a week had half the risk of heart attack and stroke! Although a similar study hasn't yet been done on women, what's good for the gander in this case is probably also good for the goose!

Orgasm also raises levels of the "feel good" chemicals in your brain and body that I talked about in Chapter 2—the neurotransmitters beta-endorphin and prolactin. If your beta-endorphin levels get too low, you're likely to overindulge in sugar, white bread, alcohol, tobacco, or drugs—"feel bad" items. And then you say to yourself, *Why did I do that?* So having sex on a regular basis not only feels good, but it also helps prevent cravings that lead to unhealthy habits and behaviors.

Increasing prolactin, the bonding hormone, increases your sense of safety and security in the world and makes you feel like you belong, which is essential for a healthy immune system. Prolactin also promotes lower blood pressure and a feeling of calm. So regular sex helps strengthen your immune system and cardiovascular system, too! Not only that, but believe it or not, it can also improve your sense of smell! This happens because increased prolactin levels cause new neurons to grow in the part of the brain that controls smell. You might even say that thanks to increased prolactin, sex helps your brain get bigger!

From an Eastern perspective, sexual energy is the same as life energy. When you can consciously increase and direct this sexual energy whether during meditation or sex itself (more on how to do this is coming up in the next chapter), it can help rebuild organs within the body. That's why sexual energy is one of the most powerful energies you have for creating health and vitality. And you don't need to have a partner to benefit—you can consciously use sexual energy all by yourself! (More on *that* in the next chapter as well!)

Good Sex Is Also Safe Sex

Please heed one very important note: Sex and sexual pleasure can enhance your health only if you're having safe sex. If you're having sex with a new partner or if your relationship isn't monogamous, it is vitally important that you protect yourself from sexually transmitted diseases, including genital herpes, genital warts, hepatitis B, and even HIV. You might not think that you're at risk for such things at this point in your life, but the fact is that the incidence of HIV among people aged 50 and up is rising twice as fast as the incidence in young adults.

True, most people who contract sexual diseases aren't over 50. Even so, 11 percent of new HIV infections happen to people in this age group—a number that's hardly insignificant. After all, any partner you have is only as safe as every partner he or she has ever had, and as safe as every partner *they* have ever had, and on and on.

I'm sharing these statistics with you not to scare you, but to empower you to take *full* responsibility for your health. And that means taking whatever steps are necessary to make sure that you don't contract something you don't want. Keep your partner's body fluids out of your vagina, anus, and mouth until you've both been tested and know each other's full status. This is the best way to show respect for yourself as well as for your partner.

When you've taken these measures and know that you can talk openly and honestly with your partner, the feeling of safety and security it will give you (as well as the increased intimacy you'll experience) will make your sexual experiences even richer. You'll see!

Sex as a Spiritual Experience

Sexual pleasure also feeds your spiritual health. Human sexuality expert Gina Ogden, Ph.D., conducted the first nationwide survey on integrating sexuality and spirituality, talking to more than 3,800 men and women over a two-year period. The data from her study, which she calls Integrating Sexuality and Spirituality (ISIS), has filled two books so far (*The Heart and Soul of Sex* and *The Return of Desire*), with a third on the way.

When Dr. Ogden asked what qualities sexuality involves in their lives, 83 percent of those who answered the survey said oneness with a Higher Power. In addition, she reports that almost half (47 percent) said that they'd experienced God at the moment of sexual ecstasy (which may or may not mean orgasm).

Remember that when you experience sexual pleasure, you're doing far more than just having a good time. You're actually invoking the Sacred Feminine and allowing that energy to live and grow (and sometimes even explode) inside of you. In a sense, sexual pleasure is a way of breathing life into your own sacredness while at the same time, that sacredness is breathing life into your physical body.

When you actively seek to enhance your experience of joy and pleasure on a daily basis, you can feel your life force growing and expanding. This results in enormous health benefits on all levels: physical, emotional, and spiritual. You program your body for better health every time you accept pleasure—sexual and otherwise—into your life.

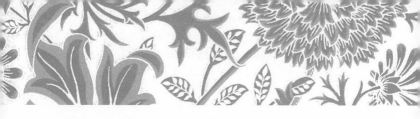

CHAPTER FIVE

The 7 Secret Keys That Will Open the Door to Wonderful Sexuality and Sensuality after Menopause

The path to great sex and enhanced pleasure after menopause can be summed up in seven keys that you'll discover as you read on. You don't necessarily have to follow them in order, and you may even want to use more than one key at a time. In fact, I highly encourage it! You may find some easier than others, and you may not want to take each and every suggestion I offer. Nevertheless, I assure you that some version of each key is vital for your maximum pleasure and vibrant health—not to mention a dynamite sex life. So try to stay open, dive right in, and have *fun* finding what works best for you!

1. Become an Ardent Explorer of Your Own Pleasure

Pay attention to what delights, inspires, and uplifts you. Remember that whatever you pay attention to expands! So if you're focusing on what pleases you, you're going to get more of it. (And conversely, if you're spending a lot of time thinking about what you feel you lack or what you don't like about your life, guess what will happen? You'll get more of that negative stuff back!)

Be as specific as possible, and write down everything you think of. I want you to really have fun with this! And then look for ways to make those desires manifest. The idea is to cultivate more joy, moment by moment. For example, one of my big pleasures is taking a hot bath each evening. Whenever I travel, I insist on a room that has a tub instead of just a shower. There's something about immersing myself in water that's very healing; it restores me in a way that nothing else does.

Do you like sexy lingerie? Go shopping for something new—and then wear it! Not just sometimes—wear it regularly. (It won't bring you nearly as much joy if it's just sitting in your bureau drawer!) Do you enjoy curling up with a book, but seldom make the time to read? Either wake up 15 minutes earlier each day to read, or if you're not a morning person, commit to going to bed with your book 15 minutes early every evening. If you love fresh flowers, don't wait for someone to send them to you. Buy some for yourself once a week—even if it's just a bouquet you pick up in the florist's section of the grocery store while you're doing your weekly food shopping. Better yet, call in an order and have a glorious bouquet delivered with a love note to yourself.

If you love getting a massage, make an appointment for one at least once a month. If you can't afford that, agree to exchange a back rub or foot rub with your partner or best friend on a regular basis. You can do the same with a manicure or pedicure.

Maybe you'd like a romantic evening out with your partner on a regular basis. (Who wouldn't?) Ask for it! And be very specific about what would please you. You'll be surprised how willing your partner will be to help make it happen once you request it. (If you don't believe me, just try it. What do you have to lose?) Even if the two of you just go for a drive together to look at the stars on a warm summer night, you'll be cultivating more joy.

Some other ideas you might put on your list include the following: going to the movies more often, hiking or taking a very long walk once a month, finally learning how to play a musical instrument, calling an old friend you haven't talked to in a long time but think of often, enrolling in an adult evening class, joining a book club, taking up a sport, or orchestrating a monthly girlfriends' lunch or dinner. I once decided to take Argentine tango lessons with some friends, and we had a blast. Talk about romantic and sexy!

I know a woman who changed her whole morning mind-set when she simply started hitting the snooze button on her alarm clock—a small indulgence that she'd never allowed herself to take before. She had to set her alarm ten minutes earlier, but instead of a negative thought being the first thing to pop into her head each morning as she heard the drone of the alarm, her first thought now became an indulgent, *Ah . . . I can turn that horrible noise off and lie here for ten more minutes, enjoying my comfortable bed.* And then that positive feeling set the tone for her whole day. Get the picture?

Think Big

Attracting small things that please you is great— in fact, it's wonderful! I want you to do lots of that. But why stop there? I encourage you to really go for it. While you're making your list, resist the temptation to limit yourself to what you think is possible or even probable. Don't edit your desires. Take note of the smaller things, but include all the big things, too—even if you think they're not likely to come your way anytime soon.

The truth is when you think big, *big things happen.* Here's why: When you save a little money, you can accomplish only small projects with it. But when you save big bucks, you can finance much bigger plans. Thinking about what you want to bring into your life is like saving money—the more you think about and envision what you want instead of what you don't want, the more ability you'll have to create it.

Desire Is the Voice of God

Trust your deepest desires and you'll soon be watching them unfold. Believe it or not, the universe wants to make you happy. It's rigged that way. Your specific desires are, in fact, the language God/Goddess/Your Higher Power/Source Energy uses to speak directly to you in order to tell you what will bring you maximum fulfillment. As long as they don't bring harm to you or another person, these ideas aren't guilty pleasures. True, sustainable pleasure and passion are directives from a higher source, so don't knock them. Go enjoy!

Yet all too often, women are afraid to connect with their desires because they feel like they're acting selfishly. They also feel guilty for wanting something or that they don't deserve to have what they long for. If this describes you at all, I want you to know this: Getting in touch with your specific desires and then manifesting them isn't just good for you, it also uplifts the entire planet. That's right! The more you get in touch with what you really, really want and then make it happen, the more you end up giving to everyone else around you—and the more you free others up to go for what they want, too. And on it goes. The effects are far-reaching!

Remember, you owe your very existence to desire—desire and pleasure are what created you (and your children and everyone else you love) in the first place. You were conceived with an orgasm (at least your father's orgasm). The entire universe, in fact, started with a big bang!

I'm sure there are some of you out there who are pretty satisfied with your life right now and feel that you already cultivate a fair amount of pleasure and joy. That's terrific. Bravo! But that's still not going to get you off the hook. I want to challenge you to cultivate even *more* joy. That's right—look more closely, search deeper, and find more things that will help you keep dialing up the pleasure, because the fact is that human beings are designed to experience unlimited pleasure and joy (which are available to each of us in an infinite supply). You're always capable of experiencing more pleasure than you currently allow yourself to feel. So no matter where you are on the joy scale at the moment, get busy and ramp it up. Your health and happiness depend on it!

2. Turn Yourself On!

This step is all about rewiring your brain and body for receiving maximum pleasure. Remember, the brain is the biggest sex organ in the body! Your sexuality involves infinitely more factors than merely what happens with your genitals.

Women with spinal-cord injuries who can't feel anything below their waist are still capable of having orgasms because their brains are able to receive signals of sexual response through alternative pathways. Sex researcher Gina Ogden, Ph.D., reported in her book *Women Who Love Sex* that some women are able to climax from merely *thinking* about what erotically stimulates them. This is true because sexual response is related to your total being—your physical, emotional, psychological, and spiritual self.

This means that you can learn to *turn yourself on* by consciously choosing thoughts and behaviors that will not just allow, but will actually encourage, your body, mind, and spirit to feel younger, sexier, and more alive. You can turn yourself on whether or not you're already having sex regularly, whether you have a partner, or whether you even think it's possible to do so. If you have a body and a brain and you're still breathing, you can get in touch with your sexuality and sensuality, and learn to turn yourself on.

Turning On Also Involves Turning Off

The turn-on first requires reprogramming your brain to switch on positive, life-affirming thoughts. It also requires switching *off* the ways of thinking that keep you from feeling the full charge of your life force—thoughts such as *I'm too old for that, I'm too heavy to be sexy, I'm not pretty anymore,* and *I don't have the energy for great sex.* Because you've most likely been running these old, self-limiting programs for quite some time, it may take a lot of effort to switch to new thoughts that will bring you more joy and greater amounts of life force. Be patient.

The key is not to judge yourself or beat yourself up for the old patterns. In fact, as soon as you do so (such as thinking, *There I go again, I'll never be able to program my thoughts!*), you're reinforcing *more* negative thinking. The secret is that as soon as you notice the old thoughts floating through your mind, simply love yourself for having them by saying something like, "I'm so adorable for having these thoughts. And how lovely that I have the power to change them." Then immediately focus your attention on whatever new thought patterns will bring you maximum pleasure.

For example, when you catch yourself thinking, *I hate these flabby old thunder thighs. Yuck! Who could love these?* immediately change your thinking to: *I love having my thighs caressed, and my partner loves having me wrap my thighs around him when we make love. Yum!* Out with the old automatic thoughts about your thighs, and in with the new, more positive and pleasurable thoughts.

I must warn you—this isn't easy at first, and it may seem silly. But it *does* work. Trust me and don't give up. Start switching your focus with your next negative thought, and then build from there. If you slip up, just start again. The more you consciously make this change, the more positive, life-affirming, nitric oxide–stimulating thoughts will start circulating in your mind to turn on your body. Once that happens on a regular basis, you'll find it infinitely easier to keep choosing the positive thoughts until eventually, they become your new dominant thought patterns.

The reason why this works is because loving, pleasurable thoughts connect you directly with your life force. It's like sowing seeds and then watering and tending them until they yield a bountiful crop. Negative, hopeless, and critical thoughts, on the other hand, drain your life force. The effect is like never watering those plants and keeping them from getting sunshine—they eventually wither and die. Don't let that happen any longer!

This positive mind-set is vitally important because it's absolutely necessary to value and respect yourself enough so that you *want* to turn yourself on and believe that you *deserve* the turn-on. If you need a little help with this, imagine that you're a visiting dignitary, a well-loved and highly revered celebrity, or even a goddess—any figure that, in your mind, would deserve pleasure and special consideration. Imagine how you'd be treated if you were that woman, and then treat yourself that way!

Ladies, Start Your Engines!

A great way to immediately experience the power of your own sexuality and sensuality is to use affirmations that really light your fire. A few good examples include:

- *I make love with unleashed abandon. I am an unbridled, gorgeous, sexy force of nature.*

- *I am Aphrodite incarnate. My body, mind, and spirit are wide-open channels for total sexual ecstasy.*

- *I am completely turned on and irresistible.*
  I am the embodiment of wild abandon and
  pleasure. I am the Divine courtesan.

- *Divine love and Divine sexuality now*
  awaken me to sexual pleasure beyond my
  wildest dreams.

Write some affirmations of your own, focusing on words and phrases that appeal specifically to you. Choose one and say it out loud to yourself at least twice a day. Then watch how your body responds as your nitric oxide levels soar.

Remember that sexuality is a total sensory experience, involving your whole body and all five senses. Sight, sound, taste, feel, and scent can play a pivotal role in the turn-on. Get creative and experiment with what works for you. The following suggestions each involve at least one, if not two or more, of the senses:

— Read books that you find at least somewhat erotic. It could be anything from classic bodice-ripping romance novels (I love *The Wolf and the Dove* by Kathleen E. Woodiwiss, as well as her other books) to erotica written especially for women (such as the collections of erotic short stories edited by Lonnie Barbach, Ph.D.). Anaïs Nin's erotica *(Delta of Venus and Little Birds)* is also an excellent choice. Do you know why 80 percent of books published today are romance novels? It's because they turn women on. A friend of mine calls them *cliterature!*

— Watch more sensual movies (with or without your partner). For most women, the movies with the highest turn-on potential are those with a good sound track, a good story, and good lighting. (Hardcore porn is a big turnoff for me and for many other women.) A few suggestions include *Wild Orchid, Emmanuelle, Emmanuelle II,* and *Two Moon Junction.*

Whatever erotic or sensual films you watch (or books you read, for that matter), make sure they aren't degrading to women in any way. Tapping into your sensuality should help build your self-esteem, not tear it down.

— Redecorate your bedroom to make it more sensual. Pick paint colors and fabrics that suggest warm flesh tones such as pinks, peaches, ivories, and beiges. Buy the finest sheets you can afford, use lighting that flatters skin tones, and make sure that the space is restful and inviting. (That means eliminating things such as a desk where you pay bills, exercise equipment, and most definitely your computer!)

— Try a little aromatherapy. Light scented candles or burn incense. Use scented massage oils—some are even flavored! Wear perfume or cologne even when you're not going out (and wear different scents for different moods). Tuck a fragrant sachet in your underwear drawer.

— Play music that gets you in the mood. This could be soft and sweet (such as love songs or folk classics by artists like James Taylor), or it could be something wild with a driving beat (like any great dance music). You might even try playing a selection of oldies that were popular when you were young—but choose those that you have a positive association with and that will remind you of good times. Another option is to play a CD with nature sounds—many women find ocean waves or the sound of rain especially sexy.

— Wear sexy lingerie (even if you're sleeping alone) and wear sexy underwear (even if you're just going to work or the grocery store that day). It feels divinely sensual to walk around knowing you have that kind of secret!

— Take sensual baths by candlelight, either with bubbles or scented oils, with music playing in the background. Use rich, creamy, scented body lotion after every bath or shower. Find ways to enjoy touching and caressing your body that are sensual but not necessarily sexual.

— Fantasize more often. You don't have to imagine a steamy X-rated scene—but kudos to you if you do! All you need to visualize is something that makes you feel sexy and alive. You might fantasize about wearing a sexy dress and walking into a room full of people, flirting with a good-looking guy, sunbathing on the beach in a daring bathing suit (or maybe topless!), or even enjoying a romantic dinner with your partner (naked, of course).

Once you get started turning yourself on, you'll love how it makes you feel. And you'll soon come up with many more ideas on your own. Remember that if you can dream it, you can achieve it. Your body can't tell the difference between fantasy and reality. And it will respond with perfect "turn-on" to the hot thoughts you're thinking—every time!

3. Remember That a Turned-on Woman Is Irresistible!

Your desire—your ability to get turned on—is virtual Viagra for your partner. There is no more potent aphrodisiac on the planet than a woman who feels irresistible. Talk about a position of power! When you feel deliciously sexy (whether or not you currently have a partner), you exude life force and enthusiasm that is positively contagious! For example, I've met more than one woman whose husband no longer experienced erectile dysfunction after she allowed herself to feel more pleasure in her life.

As a woman, *you* are the keeper and the source of the turn-on! Whenever *you* feel attractive and sexy, *he* (or she, depending on sexual preference) will find you attractive and sexy. It's that simple. But for this to happen, you must feel that you're turning yourself on for *you,* not for anyone else. If you're doing it for someone else, what you say and do won't ring quite as true—and it won't work as well. Only when you're turning yourself on for your own pleasure and benefit are you able to produce the kind of high-voltage, magnetic sexual energy that brings you the best sex you've ever had in your life.

The reason why women are the keepers of the turn-on is because we have a global response to life force wherever we see it. For example, recent research shows that women experience increased blood flow in their genitals when they view couples having sex—any couples (heterosexual or gay couples of either sex). Men, on the other hand, have a sexual response watching two women or a woman and a man, but only if they're gay or bisexual do they respond to watching two men having sex. This doesn't mean that the women in the study are bisexual or lesbian simply because they're turned on by the life force of sex in both genders (not that there's anything wrong with that, as Jerry Seinfeld would say). It does mean that wherever women see life force being played out, we resonate with it as if we were tuning forks. Women—including you!—are the very source of desire.

Scientific evidence supports this. Researchers have found that when a woman is ovulating, for example, her egg sends out a chemical signal that attracts sperm to it. Women also emit pheromones (odorless molecules secreted by glands in the armpits and pubic area) that make them more attractive to men during ovulation. You could say that women possess a type of chemical magnetism, a subtle force that makes people want to be around them.

What's more, this force isn't limited to sexual attraction. Everyone around you feels the tug. (You probably see this in your own kids or those of family members—children always seem to prefer their mothers in general, and they definitely gravitate to them more than to their fathers when they're upset or stressed.) Women's power of attraction is positively primal!

Who, *Me?*

Most women have no idea how much power they truly wield in this area. Our culture supports women in constantly comparing themselves to what society deems beautiful and sexy, and then feeling subpar when they decide that they don't measure up. Another unspoken rule in our culture is that every woman who is worth anything has a man, so if you don't have a partner, you're obviously undesirable. That's absolutely laughable! There's only one person on the planet who needs to see you as vibrantly sexy—*you*. Once you see yourself as that unbridled, gorgeous, sexy force of nature that I talked about in the last section (remember your affirmations?), others won't help but see you that way, too.

More than one man has told me that he'd be much more attracted to an overweight, plain-looking woman who talks, moves, and dresses as if she's the hottest thing going than with a model-gorgeous woman who's insecure about her looks or is otherwise just not all that fun to be with. That doesn't mean you have to walk around half naked, acting like sex on a plate to get noticed. I'm talking about your goddess persona here, not your tramp potential.

But don't just take my word for it. See for yourself with this fun exercise: Think of an actress or even a favorite character in a book who has a sexy side to her. Then, for an afternoon or evening, pretend you're that person—walk like her, talk like her, and even think like her. You might even try dressing a little like her just to make it easier to keep the feeling going. Do your regular errands, go out to eat, or just take a walk. Notice other people's reactions as you interact with them (or even just pass them on the street). You just might surprise yourself!

Exposing the Secret

I'm sure you've heard the saying "If you've got it, flaunt it!" Well, we've *all* got it—yourself included. And if you're not going to flaunt what you've got, then no one else is ever going to do it for you. Don't keep yourself a secret any longer. Expose yourself (metaphorically speaking, of course)!

Forget about trying to become what you think everyone else (or at least members of the sex that you're attracted to) wants you to be. Celebrate who and what you are. If you're tall, be proud of your height; don't wear flats and slump. If you have more meat on your bones than you'd like to have, consider capitalizing on your assets by say, showing off your cleavage a little.

The point is that when you make the most of what you have, instead of walking around as if you're apologizing for your perceived shortcomings or hiding what you've got, it changes everything—in a good way. Your conversation is wittier and saucier, and you laugh more often. Your face looks friendlier, and you're more approachable—you have more fun. So go for it!

When you aren't hiding from yourself (and everyone else), you're more interested in and interesting to people around you—men *and* women. In short, when you're turned on to yourself, the world turns on to you; and men (and also a lot of women) will find you incredibly intoxicating whether you're a size 6 or a 16. (Remember, by today's standards, even Marilyn Monroe would be considered a bit hefty. And who would *ever* say that she didn't exude sex appeal?)

Delicious Dialogue

Now that you've turned both yourself and your mate on, here's a little tip for what happens next. To have gloriously fabulous sex, you have to *keep yourself* turned on. Don't automatically pass that responsibility to your partner just because you're now between the sheets. Men in particular feel enormous pressure to perform, as our culture dictates that they know exactly what to do to satisfy women every time. No wonder so many men have erectile dysfunction!

Here's a tip: Take the guesswork out of it for him. Tell your partner what you like and ask for what you want—or at least give him feedback about what he's doing right. Sex is infinitely steamier with a little direction. Now isn't the time to be shy! Far from being insulted, your partner will revel in this information like it was a hot stock tip (and hopefully find it more gratifying). Knowing that he's bringing you to the brink of total ecstasy (and beyond) is an *incredible* turn-on for him.

Of course, in order to tell your mate exactly what you want and how you want it, you have to know yourself. You're in the best position to train your partner to be a good lover when you know your own body's sexual likes and dislikes intimately, which brings us to the next section. Ready to dive in? Good! But forget about your bathing suit . . . for this next section, ladies, we're going skinny dipping!

4. Practice Makes Pleasure!

You can't expect your partner to know how to please you sexually if you don't know how to please yourself. He (or she) wasn't born knowing exactly what you need in bed. For that matter, neither were you! This is acquired knowledge; it's not all instinct, so don't attempt to guide another person through territory that you've never personally ventured into yourself. Let the exploration begin!

As Jocelyn Elders, M.D., the first African-American surgeon general, once said (on television, no less): "We know that more than 70 to 80 percent of women masturbate, and 90 percent of men masturbate, and the rest lie."

I want to say right off the bat that I hate the word *masturbation*. It has such heavy, shameful connotations. I prefer the term used in ancient Taoist literature: *self-cultivation*. Self-cultivation and self-pleasuring imply nothing but positive growth, delight, amusement, and satisfaction.

What it all comes down to, however, is practice. It's the only way you can discover what really turns you on. Self-cultivation is how you learn to put the key into your own ignition, as Regena Thomashauer (Mama Gena) puts it. It's how you rewire yourself for maximum pleasure and nitric oxide production. And it's an empowering *health* practice—just like meditating or exercising. In addition to just plain feeling good, regular self-pleasuring also keeps your vagina well lubricated and enhances blood flow to the pelvis. Nipple stimulation even enhances breast health. So practice on a regular basis—twice a week, at least!

The Power of Breath

Breath is vitally important to cultivating your sensual and sexual energy because it helps circulate pleasurable feelings throughout your whole body, enabling you to feel them fully. Eventually, you'll be able to consciously move that life-force energy around your body at will, just by using your breath and intent. During sex (with yourself or with your partner), you can even direct orgasm throughout your entire body, allowing it to fill every organ and sink into your bones. Wow!

To start understanding how this works, I recommend that you try the following breathing exercises, based on ancient Taoist principles. The Tao (pronounced "dow") is a Chinese term that translates as "the way" and refers to the way in which the universe is ordered and how energy flows in the natural world. Many such practices have traditionally been available only to a select few—although more recently, they've been openly discussed and taught not only in Asia but also all over the world. In my experience, women who practice these techniques have a timeless energy and an unusually youthful appearance.

The following exercises that I'd like to share with you are taught by Saida Désilets—the founder of The Désilets Method, which is a program that's dedicated to the education and empowerment of sexual energy. (All of these exercises and more are detailed in Saida's book, *Emergence of the Sensual Woman,* as well as in her DVD, *Tao of Ener'chi*—both of which I highly recommend. For more information, see Saida's Website: **www.thedesiletsmethod.com**.)

Begin by simply closing your eyes and breathing slowly and deeply into your belly (and not just filling the top of your lungs, as most of us usually do). Relax into the sensation of breathing, becoming aware of your whole body drinking in life energy with each breath. Sit with this for a while and enjoy it.

Then as you go about your day, think about expanding all your senses throughout your body, just as you did with your breath. When you eat, don't just taste the food with your tongue, feel all of you—right down to your toes—tasting it. When you see something beautiful, imagine that your whole body, not just your eyes, is taking in the sight. Do the same with the sense of smell, allowing scents not to merely linger in your nose but to penetrate your very skin.

Once you're aware of your breath and how intimately connected it is to your sensuality and sexuality, you're ready to begin learning to access, harness, and circulate your sexual energy. In doing this, you awaken your nervous system by moving your awareness through a specific pathway known as the microcosmic orbit. The orbit runs from your perineum (the part of your body between your vagina and your anus) up your spine, through your head, and down the tongue and the front of your body, back down to your perineum (see the diagram on the following page).

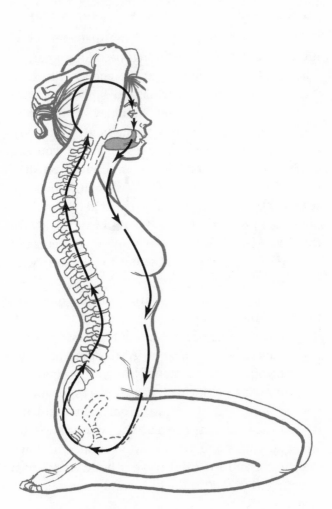

© Christiane Northrup, M.D.
Illustrated by Mark Hannon

Placing your tongue on the roof of your mouth connects this orbit. Do so, and then as you inhale, visualize a golden ball of life-force energy moving up your spine toward your head. Hold your breath for just a moment, picturing the energy spiraling like a top in your brain. As you exhale, visualize the energy moving down the front of your body as you complete the orbit.

When the energy reaches your navel, you can choose to either spiral it around and then store it there like a precious pearl for future use, or you can keep the circuit going and send it back to your perineum.

When you first try this, set aside time when you can fully concentrate on the orbit and get the energy moving. Later you can do it anywhere and any time, as often as you remember. With practice, as you awaken your life force more and more, you'll actually be able to feel the energy flowing. It's amazing!

This orbit harmonizes and balances your body and enhances your experience of orgasm. (Think of it as seeing through a window that was previously covered with a dingy film that's just been cleaned until it sparkled.) The more you practice this, the more fun all kinds of pleasure (including orgasm) will be!

THE SECRET PLEASURES OF MENOPAUSE

The Six Healing Sounds

Saida also teaches a practice called the Six Heal-ing Sounds (based on the wisdom of Taoist master Mantak Chia's Universal Tao) that helps to trans-form stressful, negative feelings into more positive, life-enhancing emotions (which, in turn, give you more access to your sensual, sexual energy). The fol-lowing are sounds you can make and exercises you can do to help you enhance the effect. With each exercise, make the sound on the exhale:

- *Hsssssssss (lungs):* With your arms above your head, turn your palms up and look up. Imagine that you're breathing in courage and self-confidence; and then as you exhale, visualize breathing out sad-ness and self-criticism, remembering to make the hsssssssss sound.

- *Choooooooo (kidneys):* With your hands on your knees, round your back and face straight ahead. Breathe in gentleness and calmness, and then while making the sound, breathe out fear and doubt.

126

- *Shhhhhhhh (liver):* Clasping your hands overhead, palms outward, lean to the left and look up. Breathe in kindness and self-acceptance, and then exhale anger and frustration.

- *Hahhhhhhhh (heart):* Use the same position as the previous exercise, but lean to the right this time. Breathe in love, joy, and respect; then breathe out hastiness, impatience, and apathy.

- *Hoooooooooo (spleen):* Press your fingers inward under your front left rib cage, and then lean forward into your fingers. Breathe in openness and fairness, and then breathe out stress and worry. (When you make this sound, do it in a guttural way, constricting your throat muscles slightly.)

- *Sheeeeeeeee (the body's thermostat):* Starting with your hands above your head, imagine that you're pressing a rolling pin down the entire length of your body. Press straight down with your palms from your head to your hips, and end with your fingers pointing down toward the ground. Breathe in a sense of radiant vitality; and breathe out any excess heat and old, sick energy.

The Inner Smile

The final simple yet powerful Universal Tao exercise that Saida has adapted specifically for sexual-energy cultivation that I'll share with you is called the Inner Smile. It helps you create a nurturing relationship with yourself, deepening your capacity for intimacy.

Close your eyes and remember the smile of someone you love and trust. As you feel yourself responding to this smile, direct your own smile into your body. Imagine that you're smiling into each of your organs and every part of your body (including your heart and genitals)—especially those parts that you don't feel very loving toward. (I recommend putting your left hand over your heart and your right hand over your genitals while doing this exercise, consciously sending the loving energy of your "high" heart to your "low" heart—your genitals.)

This exercise is extremely healing and positively transformative. As you're able to smile into each part of yourself and sense your own innate respect and joy for who you are, you'll be tapping into the limitless potential of your pleasure. This is a potent way of honoring women's greatest source of shame and turning it into your greatest source of pleasure.

To Know Thy Clitoris Is to Love Thy Clitoris

While many areas of your body may well be extremely sensitive (the lips and nipples are exquisitely erogenous, for example), your clitoris is undoubtedly the key to your sexual satisfaction, as it's the seat of all orgasms. Despite what you see in the movies and on television, less than 25 percent of women climax through intercourse alone.

The first thing you should know about this fabulous little organ is that it responds to kind words, such as telling it that it's beautiful. So talk to yourself. Look at your genitals in the mirror and tell yourself how gorgeous and sexy you are. If you say it, your clitoris will *feel* it—and so will you!

Using a lubricant (K-Y Jelly or Sylk both work really well), try stroking your clitoris while paying attention to the kinds of strokes (fast or slow, hard or gentle, back and forth, or around in circles) that bring you the most pleasure, and in what order. Search for the specific spot on the clitoris that's the most sensitive—for most women, it's on the left side at about the 1:00 position (that's *your* 1:00, looking down at yourself). So practice with this spot until you know it really, really well.

The opening of the vagina has many pleasurable areas as well. Explore your entire vulva—vagina, clitoris, labia (the lips around your vagina)—as well as your thighs, breasts, and every other part of your body. With time you can actually rewire your body for maximum pleasure simply by being present to feeling fully. For example, the upper lip and the clitoris have a direct connection in women (which is why kissing is so pleasurable). Try running your tongue or index finger over your upper lip while thinking about or touching your clitoris. There's also a rich connection between your breasts and clitoris. (Nipple stimulation enhances sexual pleasure and increases blood flow to the genitals.)

Try different touches—maybe consider stroking your whole body lightly with a soft feather. What feels good . . . and what feels *fabulous?* Find out!

Fantasizing is always a great way to dial up your excitement during self-cultivation (or during sex with a partner). Don't hold back—a fantasy, after all, doesn't have to be something that you'd actually be willing to do. One of the most productive fantasies is simply imagining yourself as deliciously sexy and irresistible. (And I'll let you in on what I hope is no longer a secret for you: That's no fantasy—*that's reality!*)

For still more luscious ideas on self-pleasuring, I highly recommend the book *The Illustrated Guide to Extended Massive Orgasm* by Steve Bodansky, Ph.D., and Vera Bodansky, Ph.D.

Getting Acquainted with Your G-Spot

Although the subject of the G-spot has been hotly debated, I assure you that it does indeed exist. This is a nickel-sized area located about two inches inside the front wall of the vagina, about halfway between the pubic bone and cervix. When you're aroused, this area swells, making it easier to find—especially if you kneel or squat and then feel for it with your fingers. You may find it easier to have multiple orgasms by stimulating this spot, so practice with it! (By the way, some experts say midlife women get more pleasure from G-spot stimulation because their lower estrogen levels make their vaginal lining thinner, which in turn makes the G-spot more prominent.) The G-spot is called the "sacred spot" in Tantra because it is felt to be the center of a woman's Shakti or goddess power.

For detailed instructions, read *The G Spot and Other Recent Discoveries about Human Sexuality* by Alice Kahn Ladas, Beverly Whipple, and John D. Perry. To learn more about the sacred spot and Tantra, I highly recommend *Tantra: The Art of Conscious Loving* by Charles and Caroline Muir.

Have fun with these ideas, and practice them regularly. As you experiment, you'll find that your physical body is capable of unlimited pleasure—you simply can't be *too* good to yourself. You'll also see that your ability to experience joy on all levels will increase. So have a blast!

5. Recognize and Release Anger and Negativity

Anger, resentment, and doubt are the enemies of turning yourself on. If you want to keep feeling deliciously sexy and desirable, you must make a habit of choosing to experience pleasure—and that means consciously letting go of your negative emotions. You can't feel pleasure *and* negativity at the same time. Believe me, the blood won't go where it's supposed to go (to your genitals), and the turn-on just turns off.

After all, no fire can continue burning if you stop feeding the flame and douse it with water. Hanging on to your anger by brooding over your frustration and why it's justified is like covering your fabulous feminine flame with a bucket of cold water. All you're left with then is a chill!

I'm not saying that you should be Suzy Sunshine all the time—that's not realistic. Experiencing a full range of emotions is a vital part of vibrant health, but what *isn't* healthy is getting stuck in negative emotions over the long term. Feel the emotion when it comes, use it constructively and effectively to change whatever is needed, and then move on. And as you do so, *let go* of the anger, doubt, or resentment—whatever it may be—and you'll feel so much better.

Remember that this is a process, not an event. You'll probably have the opportunity to let go of negativity at least several times each day. As often as possible, ditch what keeps you feeling bad and make the more empowering choice.

Expect Resistance

One of the most effective tactics for dealing with negativity is to expect it. As soon as you decide to bring more joy and pleasure into your life, anger, grief, frustration, guilt, judgment, or doubt always seems to show up to test your resolve.

Have an exit plan ready for your negativity so you don't get stuck in it (or so that *it* doesn't get stuck in *you*) when it surfaces. Call a friend, go for a walk, play with your dog, watch a good movie, or even put on some great music and dance around the room. Or go have an orgasm—that will change your focus pretty quickly! The idea is to do things that make you feel *good* and that keep your energy moving instead of becoming stuck and stagnant. In order to feel good when you're feeling bad, you must actively invite pleasure in.

With some experiences (such as divorce or death), you have to stay with your feelings for a while before you can truly release them—as the saying goes, you must feel it to heal it. So experience your grief, your anger, your sadness. Dance with them and honor them; don't sugarcoat them. But then find ways of bringing joy and pleasure into your life as you work things out. Be good to yourself, *especially* when you're dealing with something difficult. You'd do the same for your best friend, wouldn't you? Have the same regard for yourself.

Be aware that grief and fear often hide underneath other emotions—such as anger—so don't be afraid to feel your emotions all the way down to their roots. For example, it's usually much easier to be angry with individuals because of how they've hurt you or let you down than it is to feel sadness about the situation. So when you recognize and then let go of *both* your anger *and* your grief, you're healing yourself not just on the surface but from your deepest points out.

What happens next is nothing short of a miracle. When you give up the negativity, light streams in to fill the void. The more negativity you can let go of (by getting to the root of your feelings and then releasing them), the more light can come in and the more joy you're able to experience. I guarantee it!

By the way, also beware of negative pleasure. We all have a certain fascination with negative news, especially if it's about someone else! That's what feeds the tabloids. Catch yourself engaging in this energy-depleting habit (it's like nasty gossip), and stop as soon as you realize it!

Dealing with Self-Doubt

Not all negative emotions are big and splashy like anger and grief. More subtle negativity, such as self-doubt and guilt, is just as destructive (if not more so) because it plays constantly in the background like elevator music until we learn to consciously turn it off.

One of these pieces of "elevator music" that we hear a lot is our culture's overall discomfort with anyone having "too much" fun. It's the old "no pain, no gain" school of charm rearing its ugly head in yet another guise.

I've come to the conclusion that one of the primary ways in which society keeps women down (even if it's not done consciously) is by exerting social control within families. No one is better at controlling a mother's behavior than her daughter (or the other way around). I call it the mother-daughter "chain of pain."

When a mother starts to have "too much" fun, often her daughter (especially if she's a teenager) will step in to try to stop her mom in her newly discovered sensual tracks through shaming words or deeds. She may criticize the way that her mother dresses or act embarrassed by her behavior. And because we care so deeply about what our daughters think of us—and we so want their love and respect—we allow ourselves to be controlled, and we shut down. This behavior is almost always completely unconscious and unexamined on the part of the daughter (or the mother, for that matter).

This happened to one of my friends who was out dancing at a club with her adult 30-something daughters. My friend was really starting to have fun when her oldest daughter said, "Mom, no one wants to see you dancing like that!" My friend instantly felt shamed and embarrassed—and promptly sat down. So much for joy!

When she shared this story with me, I told her about my theory of social control and how even though it's convenient to blame our "culture" or "society" for the oppression of women, this actually takes place right under our noses—in our own families. But it stops the minute we have the nerve to reveal it for what it is. (Remember, it takes courage to live a pleasurable, healthy life!)

I encouraged my friend to stand up for her newly discovered, sensual, joyful self and pointed out that this would create a new blueprint not only for herself, but also for her daughters. All young women desperately need to see their mothers live full, joyful, sensual, healthy lives so that when *their* time in midlife comes, they have a strong, positive role model of what's possible. This is how we all make the world a better place for everyone!

I predicted that eventually my friend's daughters would not only accept their mom's new, happier self, they'd actually end up *celebrating* with her. And that's exactly what has happened.

Shunning self-doubt no matter what its source is an act of power. It's knowing from deep within that we're worthy of the best that life has to offer, which includes reclaiming our erotic selves. In fact, our very life force depends on it!

Make Love, Not War

It's not hard to find reasons to be resentful. For example, unless you look like a supermodel or the star of a music video, chances are you have a few self-esteem issues. You may resent yourself for how you look or resent society for making you feel that way. Many women have also been the victims of physical or emotional abuse as well—often at the hands of people who supposedly love them.

But the truth is that blaming yourself, your family, men in general, or society at large won't really change anything (except for perhaps your nitric oxide level, which will plummet). The bottom line is that you're either part of the problem or the solution. And the most effective way to be part of the solution is to rise above the level of the problem. In other words, set your sights on what you know to be right and true and on what brings pleasure (making love), instead of focusing on what you see as bad or wrong or on what perpetuates pain (making war). Don't declare a truce; declare a victory—*your* victory. And end the war for good!

6. Commit to Regularly Exploring Your Body's Pleasure Potential

If you want to reclaim your sexy self, you must make a 100 percent commitment to your sensuality and sexuality. And that means nurturing this essential part of yourself on a regular basis, not merely every once in a while. You wouldn't brush your teeth every other Tuesday and expect fabulous dental health, would you? Of course not!

Do whatever it takes to see yourself as a vibrantly sexy, sensual, and desirable woman every day of your life. You'll find that by following a nitric oxide–enhancing lifestyle and using the power of positive (and sexy) thoughts and beliefs, you'll be able to train your body over time to feel more pleasure than you've ever felt in the past. In fact, there's no ceiling on the amount of pleasure you can enjoy!

For example, it's no myth that women are multi-orgasmic. Having multiple orgasms is quite possible— for *any* woman, including *you*. And because men can learn to climax without ejaculating, thus maintaining their erections, midlife men can also be multi-orgasmic.

In fact, couples trained in extended massive orgasm (EMO) can learn to reprogram their central nervous systems in order to experience orgasms lasting up to an hour! (For more information and detailed instructions on this, read the books *The Illustrated Guide to Extended Massive Orgasm* by Steve Bodansky, Ph.D., and Vera Bodansky, Ph.D.; *The Multi-Orgasmic Woman,* by Mantak Chia and Rachel Carlton Abrams, M.D.; *The Multi-Orgasmic Man,* by Mantak Chia and Douglas Abrams; and *The Multi-Orgasmic Couple,* by Mantak Chia, Maneewan Chia, Douglas Abrams, and Rachel Carlton Abrams, M.D.)

I share this with you not to make you feel pressured to be multiorgasmic, but to illustrate what's possible when you're willing to make a total commitment to nourishing and expanding your sensuality and sexuality. You'll also find that making a commitment to living life as a sexy, sensuous woman will spill over into and enhance every aspect of your health—your weight, sleep patterns, blood pressure, and even your hormone levels.

There's also evidence that many midlife women could balance their hormones naturally through exactly what I'm talking about here: opening their hearts, getting in touch with their sexuality, allowing themselves to receive pleasure, dialing up their excitement, and letting more joy into their lives. (Don't let this stop you from using bioidentical hormones if you're doing well on them, however.) The same can be true for those who rely on antidepressants to make it through the day, and on sleeping pills to endure the night. So get ready to be healthier, starting now!

Don't Just Have More Sex

If you have a partner, explore your sensuality together on a regular basis, discovering what feels good and what feels even better. Don't make it all about intercourse, as that's a limited way to express sexuality. And don't make it solely about the "goal" of orgasm, either. Just commit to feeling as much pleasure as possible—and also pay attention to where you feel all pleasurable sensations in your body. Remember, whatever you pay attention to expands.

Do things like giving each other foot or shoulder rubs, and maybe have your partner give you baths sometimes. Showering together can also be a sensual delight: Use slow, sensual strokes and bath products that smell and feel divine.

Keep the romance alive with special nights out or evenings in, dining by candlelight with music. Write each other love notes, give each other flowers, or make other gestures of genuine caring and affection. Ballroom dancing is fabulous, too. Keep thinking of new ways to connect and express your love for one another outside the bedroom. And don't save it only for Valentine's Day or your anniversary!

Add creativity and novelty to your lovemaking as well. One woman I know loves it when her partner ties a silk scarf over her eyes and then spends time just caressing her. The blindfold heightens her senses and builds anticipation because she's never sure what type of luscious caress is coming next.

Be open to different ways of pleasing each other sexually besides intercourse, including manual and oral sex. Remember that only 25 percent of women experience orgasms regularly through intercourse alone; the rest need more intense clitoral stimulation.

When you do have intercourse, experiment with different positions. I recommend the woman-on-top position, which gives the clitoris maximum stimulation. You can move however you need to so that you hit the right spot in just the right way. Also in this position, you can more easily stimulate your clitoris yourself using your fingers or occasionally a vibrator (although over time, for some women, vibrators can dull sensation, so I don't recommend using them on a regular basis).

It's also vital that you become comfortable talking about what you like in bed and giving instructions. The best way to do this is to give positive feedback every time your partner does something right—as in "Ohhh, that feels great—I'd like more of that." Believe it or not, using words and sounds heightens pleasurable sensations because of the rich connections between the brain, throat, and genitals. Making sounds and giving verbal feedback can take some practice, but it's well worth it.

At first, if you're not used to speaking this frankly and the thought of it makes you cringe, an easy way to start is by reading erotic literature together. It can be much less intimidating to read someone else's erotic words than it is to speak your own.

You'll probably find that your partner will welcome this sharing because, trust me, your partner *wants* to please you. Men may hate asking for directions when they're driving, but that's only because they tend to feel a bit threatened when they're not on top of what's happening. If you subtly guide your partner in bringing you pleasure by giving positive feedback with every stroke and every move that feels good, you'll be helping your lover to be *very* on top of things—in a totally new (and extremely intimate) way. (For more practical information, read *Mama Gena's Owner's and Operator's Guide to Men* by Regena Thomashauer, or better yet, sign up for one of her courses at: **www.mamagenas.com**.)

Such open sharing and feedback will greatly enhance any relationship, and sometimes this alone can even save a marriage! In fact, studies show that sexually assertive women (those who ask for what they want) have stronger libidos, more orgasms, and greater satisfaction with their sex lives and their relationships. (This is why I suggest never faking an orgasm. Not only is it counterproductive, but it robs you and your partner of this kind of true pleasure and intimacy.)

Taking responsibility for your own pleasure in bed is an important part of claiming and celebrating your sensual nature. When you keep reminding yourself that *you* are what makes sexual ecstasy happen for you, you'll automatically make it a regular, joyful, health-enhancing part of your life—with or without a partner. It's all up to you.

Tick Tock, Ignore the Clock

If your sex life isn't as good as you'd like it to be, it's probably because you've been too focused on the goal of reaching orgasm. During sex, are you thinking thoughts such as: *I've gotta get there, and it isn't happening fast enough . . . I know he wants me to climax, but I'm taking up too much time. What is he going to think of me? What's wrong with me? Why can't I just hit my stride already?*

Whenever you have these hurried thoughts, every one of those 8,000 nerve endings in your clitoris shuts right down! Trying to climax with those kinds of thoughts running through your head is like trying to light a match in a downpour. Remember, your goals should be sensual pleasure, intimacy, and a sense of closeness, which may or may not involve orgasm. So lighten up, forget about the clock, and learn the art of *receiving* pleasure.

Speaking of speed, there's certainly nothing wrong with having a "quickie" every once in a while. (In fact, going from zero to 95 miles per hour can be a turn-on occasionally!) But make sure that you also devote plenty of uninterrupted time to occasions when you can slow down and just enjoy the process. Train yourself to stay in the moment and bask in the delicious sensation of being touched, kissed, caressed, and loved without putting a specific goal—like reaching orgasm—on your agenda. Vera Bodansky, Ph.D., the co-author of *The Illustrated Guide to Extended Massive Orgasm*, teaches that "orgasm" begins with the first stroke. Redefining it in this way really takes the pressure off!

There is one time, however, when it's not only okay to watch the clock, it's downright recommended: when you're counting the hours or minutes to an upcoming sensual rendezvous. Get over the idea that great sex has to be spontaneous—planning for sex is very hot. Making a "playdate" allows you to look forward to it all day long. Fantasy *is* foreplay, after all!

Sensual Secret Weapons

As you become more and more comfortable making sexuality and sensuality a priority, look into what else you might do to add some zip and give yourself a bodacious boost in bed.

For example, consider having some fun with pheromones, sexual-attractant molecules secreted naturally by various glands that give off a sort of subliminal come-hither message. Reproductive biologist Winnifred Cutler, Ph.D., founder of the Athena Institute for Women's Wellness Research, was one of the first researchers to study how humans produce and respond to these chemical secretions.

After menopause, she asserts, women do secrete fewer pheromones than when they're ovulating. But don't let that dismay you. Dr. Cutler makes pheromones available commercially in a product called Athena Pheromone 10:13, which can be added directly to your perfume or cologne. Don't worry— the pheromones are odorless, so you won't notice a change in your perfume's bouquet, but you *will* notice a change in the amount of attention you get from men.

Several studies have documented this effect. In one double-blind, placebo-controlled study published in 2002 by researchers at San Francisco State University, 74 percent of women who used the product were more sexually attractive to men. Those are pretty good odds!

If you decide to experiment with pheromones, why not let your partner try the pheromone that Dr.

Cutler makes for men called Athena Pheromone 10X? See if it turns you on more! (For more information, see Dr. Cutler's Website, **www.athenainstitute.com**. I also enjoy using the pheromone products available at **www.love-scent.com**, some of which come in foil-wrapped towelettes.)

Another sensual secret weapon that I recommend every woman develop is a strong pubococcygeous (or PC) muscle. This is the muscle you contract in order to stop the flow of urine, and it's also the major muscle that contracts when you have an orgasm. Strengthening the PC muscle increases pelvic blood flow, improves vaginal lubrication, helps urinary-stress incontinence, and enables stronger orgasms. It's also exciting for your partner during intercourse.

You can begin training your PC muscle by performing simple Kegel exercises, or vaginal contractions. Saida Désilets reports that Dr. Kegel's original work suggested only a few contractions a day rather than the "3 sets of 20" that I was taught. Find a level that's comfortable for you. The idea is to get to know your pelvic-floor muscles. By the way, you can do Kegels anywhere and anytime: driving, watching TV, cooking, sitting in the bathtub, or even standing in line at a store. Don't worry—no one will know what you're doing! If you faithfully follow these exercises and think sexy thoughts during the process, you'll start to see a difference in just a few weeks, and I guarantee that you'll find working out has never been this much fun.

Another way to strengthen the PC muscle is to use cone-shaped vaginal weights that range from 15 g to 100 g. Based on ancient Chinese techniques, the method involves inserting one of the weights into the vagina and holding it in place for at least 5 minutes twice per day, gradually working up to 15 minutes twice daily. As this becomes easier, you move to the next cone, which is heavier. Most women see a difference in four to six weeks of regular use. Many physical therapists use this technique to help with urinary control issues. And in my experience, this method is very effective, particularly for urinary stress incontinence. (Google "vaginal weights" to find a source.)

Another technique that I highly endorse is the use of a jade egg (available from **www.thedesilets method.com**). Saida Désilets teaches specific exercises with the jade egg in both her book, *Emergence of the Sensual Woman*, and also on a CD of jade-egg practices.

Stop Keeping Score

While you're exploring your midlife sensuality and sexuality, remember that it's not a numbers game. Being committed to a healthy sex life isn't about having a certain amount of orgasms or sexual interludes each week. Don't confuse quantity with quality. For example, a recent study from the University of Chicago found that many couples who have intercourse only three times a month are completely satisfied with that. Good for them!

Aim for sharing true intimacy with sex instead of merely having intercourse. In our culture, women are encouraged from childhood to open their "high" hearts (the heart in our chests) and close our "low" hearts (our genitals). As a result, we tend to lead with our hearts, freely showering love and affection on our mates . . . but sometimes holding back sexually. With men, it's just the opposite: They tend to close down their high hearts and not let us in, although they're more open sexually. To experience true intimacy and great sex, men and women need to learn how to work with *both* their high hearts and their low hearts.

If a man seeks true intimacy with a woman, he has to woo her with words, attention, and affection.

Then she'll feel safe enough to surrender to him sexually. On the other hand, in order to win a man's vulnerable heart, a woman must approach him with the same tenderness that she desires from him. If she criticizes or finds fault with him, he'll protect his heart, but if she makes him her hero, then he'll feel safe enough to share his heart with her.

Saida Désilets, an expert in female sexual energy, explains that we can see this anatomically. Men's genitals are on the outside—and they lead with their sexuality (while women keep theirs hidden). On the other hand, women's breasts are on the outside—and they lead with their hearts and affection (while men's hearts, like women's genitals, are much less obvious).

To achieve vibrant health, you must commit yourself not just to having sex, but also to engaging and nurturing your sexual energy and then making love on many levels. That keeps your life energy flowing and encourages positive, caring connections with yourself, your partner (if you have one), and the rest of the world. That's the total package of mind, body, and spirit!

7. *Live Your Life in a Way That Excites, Motivates, and "Turns On" Others to Be at Their Best—and Healthiest*

When you start living your life as a totally alive, turned-on woman, an amazing thing happens: Not only does this bring you (as well as your partner, if you have one) an amazing amount of pleasure and happiness, but you also start having a positive effect on everyone else around you. In fact, your joyful outlook becomes positively contagious!

The effect is similar to what happens when you're in a good mood. You've probably often seen how your upbeat mood can put a smile on someone else's face, but the effect I'm talking about here is much deeper and more powerful than just spreading a few smiles.

When you commit to discovering, nurturing, and then living your true passion, it's as if you're stoking a fire in your soul. And you are—a fire fed by nitric oxide! Others then see you not only being confident and comfortable in your own skin, but also celebrating yourself and reaching for joy at every turn. As a result, *you* will inspire them to do the same. So eventually, they, too, begin making healthier choices that nurture their bodies, minds, and spirits—and on it goes from there!

Be a Source of Pleasure for Others

But that's just the start. Instead of merely being an example—as powerful as that can be—why not become a *source* of pleasure for others as well? You'll quickly see that this takes relatively little effort on your part, and it can be a great deal of fun.

For example, compliment others more often when they do something right. So many of us are used to getting feedback only when we do something wrong or displease someone else. Why not let people know that you appreciate what they've done right then and there? (This approach also works really well with family members, especially partners and kids.) Remember the saying "An attitude of gratitude creates a space for grace"—there's a lot of wisdom in that statement!

You can use this idea even when you have something negative to say. For example, if you're at a restaurant and your server takes too much time delivering your meal and it arrives cold, instead of being nasty about it, you could choose to say with a genuine smile, "This looks absolutely delicious, but it's a bit cold. Could you warm this up for me?" By not spewing anger, you save yourself from raising your blood pressure and having stress hormones coursing through your veins, which lower your levels of nitric oxide. And at the same time, you also inspire feelings of appreciation and trust in others, which help keep their nitric oxide levels stable, too. Not to mention the fact that people are much more likely to want to give you pleasure when you're giving them pleasure! It's a win-win.

I'm also a big believer in "drive-by" compliments. If I see a woman in public whose outfit, hairstyle, or jewelry is particularly striking, I let her know with a quick but genuine compliment. I do the same for men and children, too.

When you behave in this way, what you're really doing is starting a chain of positive emotion. The individual you compliment will most likely be genuinely touched—especially if it's someone you don't know who isn't expecting it. And then *that* person will feel better about him- or herself and will be in a better mind-set to keep the joy circulating.

The more pleasure you spread to others, the more you will feel yourself, and the more joyous and healthier the world around you will become. This works because of the Law of Attraction, which states that whatever you pay attention to expands. So by spending time focusing on joy and pleasure, you're simply calling more of it to you—and to everyone else you come in contact with as well. In a very short time, you'll start to see beauty in many forms and opportunities for pleasure wherever you go. It's an upward spiral!

Going Global

The idea of being a source of pleasure for others isn't limited to compliments and other quick, positive comments. You can actually use joy to help transform the world. Remember the old adage "If Mama ain't happy, ain't nobody happy"? The opposite is also true: When women are happy, everyone around them automatically feels uplifted, too. It's as if a wave of loving-kindness goes out from them and affects every living thing on the planet.

Let's think about this for a moment. By virtue of our biology, women are the main source of nurturing in the world, right? We nurture everyone around us—not just our kids. It's in our DNA!

So, then, can you imagine the difference it would make being nurtured by a woman who's fully alive and turned on by life, versus a woman who's just making it through the day? Women who have blossomed in midlife actually feed life force to everyone they come into contact with, whether or not they realize it.

That's why when women take the time and effort to be truly supportive of other women, the effect is so gratifying (we all know this). After all, haven't you experienced the incredibly uplifting power of being in a group of female friends? By the time the get-together is over, you almost always feel infinitely better than you did when you arrived, and you can't wait to spend time with each other again. It's no coincidence!

The world needs more beauty and light right now. The health of the planet depends upon our own happiness, joy, and pleasure to help raise the collective life force for all beings. Giving and receiving pleasure is a way of life that helps everyone and everything.

So get going! The only thing you have to lose by following your bliss is your suffering (and maybe a pound or two)—and *that* is worth celebrating.

**The 7 Secret Keys That Will
Open the Door to Wonderful Sexuality
and Sensuality after Menopause**

1. Become an ardent explorer of your own pleasure.

2. Turn yourself on!

3. Remember that a turned-on woman is irresistible!

4. Practice makes pleasure!

5. Recognize and release anger and negativity.

6. Commit to regularly exploring your body's pleasure potential.

7. Live your life in a way that excites, motivates, and "turns on" others to be at their best—and healthiest.

Afterword

So now you know the secret to a luscious, healthy, and pleasurable life, including great sex. This secret is precious and also very easily sabotaged by doubts, fears, and misconceptions. To protect you from that, I leave you with a few pages designed to boost your nitric oxide levels each and every time you read these words and feel their effect in your body. As a doctor, I'm giving you a prescription to read through the list daily!

- Your body is turned on and kept healthy by high levels of nitric oxide. Nitric oxide is, quite literally, the *spark of life* molecule and the fountain of youth.

- Your body was conceived in a blast of nitric oxide. All healthy, sustainable pleasures saturate your body and brain in life-giving nitric oxide. Orgasm is particularly potent in this regard.

- Your sexuality and orgasmic response are examples of how creative energy feels in your body. You always have access to this vital orgasmic energy and can learn to consciously direct it to heal your body and your life. You simply must be willing to allow more and more nitric oxide–boosting pleasure into your life, starting now.

- The secret to a healthy, happy, luscious life begins with thinking heartwarming, sexy, uplifting, kind, loving, and positive thoughts about yourself and others every single day. These thoughts instantly boost your nitric oxide levels.

- Other ways to boost nitric oxide include eating colorful, fresh, organically grown foods; exercising regularly; and also taking high-quality, well-balanced nutritional supplements daily.

- You're capable of experiencing unlimited amounts of pleasure because that's how your body was designed.

- Releasing old resentment, anger, and hurt regularly is an important part of setting yourself free to feel more pleasure and joy.

- The best sex with a partner always happens when there is commitment, trust, and vulnerability in the relationship.

- You must be willing to surrender to the magic of pleasure, joy, and love.

- Your pleasure and joy are healing forces that uplift and inspire everyone around you and also help heal the entire planet.

May you now have the courage to go forth and live pleasurably and joyfully—by becoming the Divine embodiment of all that is good, uplifting, empowering, and passionate.

Acknowledgments

My first three books, each more than 600 fully referenced pages, were the result of years of heroically hard work. I know the path of hard work very well, and I have a great deal of respect for it. But I also knew that it was time to try a different approach—one that was more feminine. More subtle. About a year ago, I birthed a specific desire: I wanted to write a book about how pleasure heals the physical body. I knew that the process of writing must match the subject matter. Because how you do it is what you get, I wanted the material to come to me and through me joyfully and effortlessly.

I began noodling around with ideas—and I even created a large table of contents. (Yes, I'm afraid that

I was on my way to writing a fourth magnum opus.) Then lo and behold, the universe stepped in and I miraculously connected with Dr. Ed Taub, Dr. Ferid Murad, and Dave and Deb Oliphant. Together we arrived at a most pleasurable way to fulfill all of my desires for my fourth book. And, praise the Divine, I also learned how to write a short book! Thank you, Dave, Deb, Ed, and Ferid.

I also acknowledge the following individuals:

Katy Koontz, for her brilliant editorial and organizational skills. Katy—you made this book such a pleasure to work on!

My team at Hay House: Reid Tracy; Kristina Tracy (who orchestrated the photo shoot for the cover and made it so much fun); Donna Abate; Margarete Nielsen; Jill Kramer; Christy Salinas; and Louise Hay, a most amazing mentor and way-shower, who has blazed a brilliant superhighway for me to dance down.

Charles Bush, for creating an effortless photo shoot for the cover and beyond; and Lori Sutherland, the Duchess of Finesse, for her magnificent help with the photo shoot.

Nancy Levin and her husband, Chris Rauchnot, for being such superstars at organizing speaking events.

Judie Harvey, for her enthusiasm, support, and wonderful editing skills.

Regena Thomashauer, the founder of Mama Gena's School of Womanly Arts, whose school has provided my daughters and me with the perfect laboratory in which to learn, practice, and perfect the discipline and fine art of pleasure.

Doris Cohen, Ph.D., whose spiritual counsel continues to bring my family and me so much peace and joy.

Sue Abel, for helping me create beauty and order in my home. I so appreciate you.

Janet Lambert, for keeping my finances in good order via her stellar bookkeeping skills; and Paulina Carr, for being willing to do whatever it takes to keep my organization flowing.

Chip Gray and the staff of the Harraseeket Inn in Freeport, Maine, for providing me with so many amazingly delicious, healthy meals served in such a pleasurable setting, along with some ingenious editorial suggestions when needed. Thanks, also, for providing the perfect lodgings for so many of my colleagues, friends, and family members.

The incredible, legendary Diane Grover, my CEO of Everything, who has been at my side, turning ideas into reality, for nearly 30 years. Diane, what

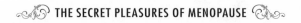

can I say? You are simply amazing and fabulous. And I'm *so* grateful.

My two daughters, Annie and Katie—who have been my biggest cheerleaders in my midlife reinvention and ongoing quest to live a life full of pleasure, joy, integrity, and abundance.

Finally, I acknowledge myself for being willing to wait until the right subject, the right format, and the right people all came together—drawn by the strength of my original Divine Desire. Ask and it is given, indeed . . . just add faith and patience.

About the Author

Christiane Northrup, M.D., is a visionary pioneer and beloved authority in the field of women's health and wellness. A board-certified ob-gyn who graduated from Dartmouth Medical School and did her residency at Tufts–New England Medical Center, Dr. Northrup was also an assistant clinical professor of obstetrics-gynecology at Maine Medical Center for more than 20 years. Recognizing the unity of body, mind, and spirit, she helps empower women to tune in to their innate inner wisdom in order to transform their health and truly flourish.

Dr. Northrup is the author of two *New York Times* best-selling books, *Women's Bodies, Women's*

Wisdom (Bantam, revised 2006) and *The Wisdom of Menopause* (Bantam, revised 2006). Her third book, *Mother-Daughter Wisdom* (Bantam, 2005), was a 2005 Quill Award nominee and was voted **Amazon.com**'s number one book of the year in both Parenting and Mind/Body Health.

Dr. Northrup has also hosted six highly successful PBS specials. Her latest, *Menopause and Beyond: New Wisdom for Women,* began airing nationwide in March 2007. Her work has been featured on *The Oprah Winfrey Show,* the *Today* show, *NBC Nightly News with Tom Brokaw, The View, Rachael Ray,* and *Good Morning America.* For more information about Dr. Northrup and her work, please visit her Website at: **www.drnorthrup.com**.

We hope you enjoyed this Hay House book. If you'd like to receive a free catalog featuring additional Hay House books and products, or if you'd like information about the Hay Foundation, please contact:

Hay House, Inc.
P.O. Box 5100
Carlsbad, CA 92018-5100

(760) 431-7695 or **(800) 654-5126**
(760) 431-6948 (fax) or **(800) 650-5115 (fax)**
www.hayhouse.com® • **www.hayfoundation.org**

Published and distributed in Australia by: Hay House Australia Pty. Ltd., 18/36 Ralph St., Alexandria NSW 2015 • *Phone:* 612-9669-4299 *Fax:* 612-9669-4144 • www.hayhouse.com.au

Published and distributed in the United Kingdom by: Hay House UK, Ltd., 292B Kensal Rd., London W10 5BE • *Phone:* 44-20-8962-1230 *Fax:* 44-20-8962-1239 • www.hayhouse.co.uk

Published and distributed in the Republic of South Africa by: Hay House SA (Pty), Ltd., P.O. Box 990, Witkoppen 2068 • *Phone/Fax:* 27-11-467-8904 orders@psdprom.co.za • www.hayhouse.co.za

Published in India by: Hay House Publishers India, Muskaan Complex, Plot No. 3, B-2, Vasant Kunj, New Delhi 110 070 *Phone:* 91-11-4176-1620 *Fax:* 91-11-4176-1630 • www.hayhouse.co.in

Distributed in Canada by: Raincoast, 9050 Shaughnessy St., Vancouver, B.C. V6P 6E5 • *Phone:* (604) 323-7100 • *Fax:* (604) 323-2600 www.raincoast.com

Tune in to **HayHouseRadio.com®** for the best in inspirational talk radio featuring top Hay House authors! And, sign up via the Hay House USA Website to receive the Hay House online newsletter and stay informed about what's going on with your favorite authors. You'll receive bimonthly announcements about Discounts and Offers, Special Events, Product Highlights, Free Excerpts, Giveaways, and more!
www.hayhouse.com®